Statistics for Biology and Health

Series Editors

Mitchell Gail
Division of Cancer Epidemiology and Genetics
National Cancer Institute
Rockville, MD, USA

Jonathan M. Samet
Department of Epidemiology, School of Public Health
Johns Hopkins University
Baltimore, MD, USA

More information about this series at http://www.springer.com/series/2848

Klaus Krickeberg • Pham Van Trong
Pham Thi My Hanh

Epidemiology

Key to Public Health

Second Edition

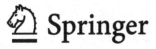 Springer

Klaus Krickeberg
Grosser Kamp 4
Bielefeld, Germany

Pham Thi My Hanh
Faculty of Public Health
Thai Binh Medical University
Thai Binh, Vietnam

Pham Van Trong
Faculty of Public Health
Thai Binh Medical University
Thai Binh, Vietnam

ISSN 1431-8776   ISSN 2197-5671   (electronic)
Statistics for Biology and Health
ISBN 978-3-030-16370-9   ISBN 978-3-030-16368-6   (eBook)
https://doi.org/10.1007/978-3-030-16368-6

This Springer imprint is published by the registered company Springer Nature Switzerland AG
The registered company address is: Gewerbestrasse 11, 6330 Cham, Switzerland

In Memory of Hoang Thuy Nguyen

We had intended to dedicate this book to the Former Director of the Vietnamese National Institute of Hygiene and Epidemiology, Professor Hoang Thuy Nguyen. While working on the second edition, the sad news of his death at the age of 89 years reached us. He had been active to the end in giving advice when needed.

Hoang Thuy Nguyen, who is considered the "Father of Virology" in Vietnam, studied medicine in Hanoi and Erfurt (former German Democratic Republic). After his return to Vietnam in 1959, he joined the Department of Microbiology of the National Institute of Hygiene and Epidemiology, where he was Deputy Director from 1965 to 1974 and Director from 1974 to 1994. He built it up in very difficult times on the existing basis of the Pasteur Institute of Hanoi. He added the field "Epidemiology" to classical hygiene and its microbiological foundations and supported its vigorous development. An early and constant search for contacts with scientists all over the world was a particularly striking element of his endeavors. Epidemiology in Vietnam in theory and practice and, as a consequence, Public Health rest largely on the foundations he laid.

Preface to the Second Edition

This preface incorporates the main elements of the preface to the first edition, which appeared in 2012.

The first edition of the present book was the successor to the textbook *Lessons on Epidemiology* (in Vietnamese) that had been in use at the Medical University of Thai Binh since 1990. After a critical analysis of these "lessons," we wrote a completely new text. We did it with the following objectives in mind, which are still those of the second edition.

Firstly, we want to provide the reader with an *overview* of the whole field and not restrict ourselves to particular aspects such as methods of epidemiologic studies. Thus, we cover topics that play an important role in present-day health activities but are rarely treated in existing texts. They include the epidemiology of particular diseases, both infectious and noninfectious ones; health registers, health information systems, sample surveys, elementary statistics, and epidemiologic modelling; clinical epidemiology; and nutritional, environmental, social, and genetic epidemiology. We have also added some topics that are, in our experience, often handled wrongly in the literature and need to be elucidated. Lesson 28 gives an overview of more advanced methods and subject areas that could not be treated here. We emphasize throughout the position of epidemiology as the core of Public Health. A last Lesson (29) entitled "The Role of Epidemiology in Building Coherent Systems of Public Health," which is based on recent work of us authors, was added in the present edition.

Secondly, we have tried to give the reader a clear picture of the *fundamental ideas* that underlie the field of epidemiology and to enable her or him to recognize their role in any situation in practice. It is only by being familiar with these ideas that the right questions can be asked in real situations and the right methods can be chosen to solve practical problems. Also, when reading the report on a study, a person involved in Public Health should be able to put it into the correct framework, to extract the essentials, and to judge its significance and correctness. This is all the more important as most of them will never have an occasion of participating themselves in a major study. They will later on have to base their decisions about practical matters of Public Health on publications.

Insisting on the basic ideas will also help to lay the ground for what we should like to call "population-side teaching." This is the public health analogue to "bedside teaching" of clinical medicine; it is related to, but not identical with, "community-based teaching." Part of the training in Public Health of medical students can take place in direct contact with the population. At the same time, students can help health workers on the primary level to understand simple epidemiologic facts and to use them if possible.

Our book is not intended to teach details of techniques. When engaged in an epidemiologic study or faced with an epidemiologic problem which underlies, for example, prevention of a disease, health education, outbreak investigation, or control of infectious diseases, people must know which steps are to be taken and why, but they need not know how these steps look in detail; for that they can consult specialists or appropriate manuals.

This text will also prepare its readers to use statistical software with discernment. Since many different software packages are being employed in various institutions, we have neither recommended nor used a particular one.

Thirdly, the structure of the book is largely determined by *didactic* viewpoints, and the reader is encouraged to understand them. We did not want to start with general theory and handle applications afterwards. Instead, we have tried to place the theoretical bases at their natural places. Thus, in the beginning, that is, in Lessons 1–10, most fundamental ideas appear only in a specific concrete context. They are explained in an intuitive way, not very rigorously, but sufficiently well so that the student can understand their role. Theory and methods are then provided in Lessons 11–17 when the student has already gained some feeling about them. Finally, armed with these tools, we go back to specific problems, but again, three more theoretical and general Lessons (20, 21, and 24) are put in only later, when they are needed.

This organization also corresponds to basic differences between the epidemiologies of infectious and of noninfectious diseases. Until not long ago, epidemiologic thinking in developing countries was dominated by problems of infectious diseases, but at present, noninfectious ones play an equally important role. Modern general and rigorous epidemiologic methods were mainly developed as a response to challenges by noninfectious diseases, whereas problems of the epidemiology of infectious diseases can be handled to a large extent by more elementary tools, with the exception of mathematical modelling. Finally, and most importantly, most *curative* interventions against an infectious disease in a given community also have an indirect *preventive* effect by eliminating sources of infections; nothing of the kind exists for noninfectious diseases. Therefore, most lessons on specific infectious diseases contain a section on case management, whereas none of those on noninfectious diseases do.

The reader should note that the lessons on specific problems are determined in two basically different ways: either by the outcome variable as in Lessons 6–10 and 22–23 or by the exposure as in Lessons 25 and 26.

For didactic reasons, too, we have treated systematically only the action of a *single* exposure variable, with the exception of Lesson 21 on confounding, where we have explained everything with the help of two examples. Having understood the principle of the action of one risk factor, the reader should have no difficulty in understanding the essential ideas of the role of several exposures together as they come up in the examples of Lessons 22, 23, 25, and 26 in an informal way. Similarly, we have restricted ourselves mainly to studying *binary* exposure and outcome variables.

"Missing" topics are being listed in Lesson 28. A systematic and comprehensive history of epidemiology from its beginnings is unfortunately among them, and for a good reason, it does not yet exist.

A last important didactic viewpoint is the unity of the book. It should not, and cannot, be seen as a collection of more or less independent lessons. In particular, there are very many cross-references, considered as a didactic tool, too. We have not been afraid of being repetitive in some places.

Examples and practical work are taken from the present situation of health in Vietnam. Such a coherent setting in one specific country is seen as an advantage, not as a drawback; it is preferable to illustrations from many countries that will necessarily remain diffuse and superficial. In a sense, this text is a large case study that can easily be adapted to any other developing or transition country.

It should be clear now that our book is an introduction to epidemiology for anybody interested in this field. The basic prerequisite is secondary school training. The reader may browse through the text and select what he or she likes.

There exists of course a natural readership. It consists above all of lecturers of epidemiology at universities and equivalent training institutions. The book will enable them to compose their introductory courses by selecting the material deemed appropriate; it will also provide them with a solid foundation for more advanced teaching. Students starting to specialize in Public Health and medical students in countries like Vietnam, where the basic medical curriculum includes modules pertaining to Public Health, belong to the prospective readers, too. Staff of health institutions involved in Public Health is another important part of the natural readership.

This book is particularly suited for adoption in the first courses on epidemiology in Medical Schools and Faculties of Public Health in *developing* and *transition* countries and in workshops in these countries, taught, for example, by members of international organizations.

After the publication of the first edition of the present book, a series of books entitled "Basic Texts in Public Health" started to appear in the Medical Publishing House, Hanoi, which is edited by Klaus Krickeberg, Phan Vu Diem Hang, and Nguyen Van Son. The following volumes have come out or are being produced, all of them bilingual (Vietnamese and English):

Health Education (2014)
Population Science and Public Health (2014)
Mathematics and Statistics in the Health Sciences (2017)
Environmental Health – Basic Principles (2017)
Nutrition – The Epidemiologic Viewpoint (to appear in 2019)
Traditional and Alternative Medicine in Public Health (being written)

Bielefeld, Germany Klaus Krickeberg
Thai Binh, Vietnam Pham Van Trong
Pham Thi My Hanh

Acknowledgments

Several people read part of a first draft and made many useful comments, in particular Dinh Ngoc Sy, Le Xuan Hung, Pham Ngoc Dinh, Phan Vu Diem Hang, Vu Dinh Hai, Bernhelm Booss, Lena Striedelmeyer, Axel Ekkernkamp, Uli Schmucker, and Heiko Jahn. Nguyen Thi Thu Yen supplied technical information on specific points. Two reviewers added pertinent remarks. To all of them, we owe much gratitude.

We should like to thank the Else Kröner-Fresenius-Stiftung for its financial support during the years 2008–2016 of the project of reforming the teaching of Public Health in Medical Universities and Faculties in Vietnam. It enabled us to write the first four texts quoted at the end of the Preface above. Special thanks go to Dr. Carolin Kröner for taking a constant interest and often encouraging us. The "Switzerland-Vietnam Association" and the foundation "Medico International Switzerland" provided moral, factual, and financial support that made possible the printing of the fifth of these texts; we are grateful to them, too.

Contents

Lesson 1
The Idea of Epidemiology

This lesson should give the reader a clear idea of what epidemiology really is.

1.1 Public Health

On the 23rd February 2009, Dao Duy Anh, born on 24 September 1992, consulted the Thaí Bình General Hospital because of bad stomach pains. A physician recorded the anamnesis, examined him, diagnosed an acutely inflamed stomach and wrote prescriptions for amoxiclin, rekalate, smecta and omeprazole. Anh was cured within a few days and no follow-up by medical services was required.

The handling of this case was an example of what is commonly being called "case management". It concerned the *individual* patient Dao Duy Anh. It was a curative act. Curative treatments of this kind form the essential part of "clinical medicine", a term that was derived from the ancient Greek word for "bed" (*clinee*) and the Latin word "*medicina*" (the art of healing).

Dao Duy Anh had been vaccinated at the age of 9 months against measles. In principle, every Vietnamese baby is vaccinated against measles at the *same* age, by the *same* type of vaccine and in the *same* way. It is being done systematically in the framework of the "Expanded Programme on Immunization (EPI)". This programme concerns a whole "population", namely *all* babies having reached the age of 9 months, and not a specific individual baby. Thus it is part of "Public Health". We define indeed Public Health as follows:

Public Health is the entirety of theoretical and practical activities that are related to health and deal with populations as a whole but not specifically with their individual members.

Instead of the term "population", the word "community" is often being used. It may stand for any group of persons, for example all Vietnamese children under the age of 1 on the 14th February 2019.

© Springer Nature Switzerland AG 2019
K. Krickeberg et al., *Epidemiology*, Statistics for Biology and Health,
https://doi.org/10.1007/978-3-030-16368-6_1

Unfortunately in some countries the literal translation of the word "public" into the local language means "state-run" as opposed to "private". This may lead to confusion. Private organizations, too, can very well pursue public health activities in the sense defined above. For example some so-called non-governmental organizations do it.

Vaccinating against measles is a *preventive* act. Its purpose is to prevent measles in the vaccinated children. In addition to this *direct* effect, it also has an *indirect* effect on the entire population. It reduces the number of children that could be sources of further infections, and also reduces their *infectivity*, that is, their power of infecting others; see Lesson 5. In this way it influences what is called the "dynamics" of the transmission of the disease from one child to another within the population concerned. In particular, it prevents an *epidemic* of measles.

The word "epidemic" existed in ancient Greece and meant "epidemic disease". It was derived from the words "upon" (*epi*) and "people" (*demos*); thus, it designated "something that falls upon the population". It was therefore already at that time a concept of Public Health. The term "epidemiology" seems to have appeared first in 1802 in Spain; note that the Greek word "*logos*" signifies many things, among them "description, reason". In the beginning epidemiology stood indeed only for the "science of epidemics of infectious diseases" but gradually, starting towards the middle of the twentieth century, its meaning was broadened to include all kinds of illness, not only infectious ones. The modern definition will be given in Sect. 1.3.

1.2 Descriptive Epidemiology

We have noted that epidemiology is about illness in populations, not in individual subjects. More precisely, it is concerned with the *frequency* of diseases in various parts of the population in which we are interested, the so-called "target population". First of all:

When counting cases of a disease we need a precise case definition.

This is the subject of clinical courses but for certain specific diseases we will give a case definition in order to help the reader. For the entirety of diseases and other health problems there exists the International Classification of Diseases (ICD) whose latest (10th) revision was adopted by the World Health Organization (WHO) in 1994.

The meaning of the term "frequency" will be made precise in Sect. 1.6 and then, in a more systematic manner, in Lesson 15. We can already get a vivid impression of this concept by visiting a Commune Health Station and by looking at its "Register of Consultations". The personnel of the station uses this register when filing a weekly or monthly report to its District Health Centre. For every one of the main diagnoses occurring in the station, it calculates the number of consultations during the week or month in question with that diagnosis, for example the number of consultations leading to the diagnosis "influenza syndrome". This gives the so-called "disease spectrum" in the station for the week or month. By doing it for every month of a given year and by adding up, for each diagnosis, the corresponding figures, staff of the station obtains the disease spectrum in their station for the whole year.

However, instead of simply adding up figures for all months, we may also be interested, for a given diagnosis such as "diarrhoea", in the monthly figures themselves. If we compare them with each other, we see that they describe the "time evolution" of the frequency of the diagnosis "diarrhoea", in particular its dependency on the season. In the language of modern epidemiology, these monthly figures represent the *influence* of the *factor* "time" on the frequency of the disease as diagnosed.

In addition to the factor "time" there exist other factors whose influence on the frequency of diseases can be studied with the help of the register of consultations, namely "age", "sex" and "place of residence". From the register, one can indeed calculate disease frequencies "by age", that is, in various age groups, and analogously "by sex" and "for every village".

Policlinics and hospitals have many more and in part more detailed registers than Commune Health Stations. For example, some of them indicate the occupation of the patient; in that case we can study the influence of the factor "occupation" on disease frequencies. Like the registers of Commune Health Stations these registers provide disease frequencies that are being reported to different levels like District Health Centres, Province Health Departments, and finally to the Ministry of Health.

Every year, the frequencies are summarized in the "Health Statistics Yearbook" of the Ministry. In addition, the "Health Statistics Yearbook" gives the "mortality", that is the number of deaths, by the various causes and by some of the factors age, sex etc. This is the "Descriptive Epidemiology" for all of Vietnam. There also exists a descriptive epidemiology for geographic entities such as communes, districts, provinces, countries, regions or the whole world.

Descriptive epidemiology is the representation of disease and death frequencies by some or all of the factors age, sex, time, place and occupation. Essentially, descriptive epidemiology amounts to classical health statistics.

Classical health statistics was composed of statistics of diseases (morbidity) and statistics of deaths (mortality). It started in the seventeenth century in England in the form of statistics of the *causes* of death, a topic that is nowadays part of "Population Science" (Demography). To give a general idea we present in Table 1.1 the number of deaths by the main ten causes worldwide in the year 2016, according to the World Health Organization (WHO).

In this book we shall often describe the impact of diseases by mortalities in order to convey a first impression. However, everybody dies eventually and the *age* of death also matters. If, for example, deaths by cardio-vascular diseases would occur only at a very high age, we would not consider them a health problem of overriding importance. Moreover, death is not the only negative consequence of illness. There is also pain, inability to work or to enjoy leisure, loss of friends, loss of income and

Table 1.1 Mortality by causes in 2016 in the whole world

Cause	Number of deaths (unit: one million)
Ischemic heart disease	8.76
Stroke	6.24
Lower respiratory infections	3.19
Cronic obstructive pulmonary diseases	3.17
Cancers of trachea, bronchus, lung	1.69
Diabetes mellitus	1.59
Alzheimer disease and other dementias	1.54
Diarrhoeal diseases	1.39
Tuberculosis	1.37
Road injuries	1.34

other departures from an ideal healthy life. In order to compare this "burden" between different diseases and in different populations, several indicators have been invented that take these negative attributes into account. We shall present the "Disability-Adjusted Life Years" (DALY), which has become popular. Thus, let us focus on a specific disease C such as lung cancer in a particular target population.

Firstly, the "Years of Life Lost" in the whole target population because of premature death due to C, usually called YLL, can be found from mortality statistics where the cause of death is indicated; one uses the elementary demographic methods taught in any course on demography. The definition of "Years lived with Disability" caused by C in the entire target population, to be called YLD, is more involved. It rests on the idea that it should be the length of the period from the onset of C until death, multiplied by a "weight" coefficient w between 0 and 1 that describes *how much* disability is caused by C. A heavier weight should correspond to a larger coefficient w. Thus for lung cancer or advanced obstructive chronic bronchitis, w will be relatively large. It will even be close to 1 for a disease that is crippling the patient almost completely like amyotrophic lateral sclerosis (Charcot's disease). By contrast, if C just causes minor inconveniences like a small finger lost in an accident, w will be close to 0. To determine w concretely as a specific number is a complicated affair based on subjective appreciations of the disabling effect of C in a sample of persons.

Finally, the DALY is defined as,

$$DALY = YLL + YLD.$$

This represents the disability-adjusted life years *lost* due to death and disability caused by C in the target population. One defines analogously the DALY for a whole group of diseases or even for *all* ailments together.

Typical applications of the DALY or similar indicators have been comparisons of the burden due to different diseases, or of all infectious diseases on the one hand and non-infectious ones on the other. However, like any indicator that tries to summarize the effects of many components and to represent them by a single number, the DALY is of limited usefulness. Moreover, its definition contains arbitrary elements both in YLL and in YLD. It has therefore been fairly controversial.

Until recently infectious diseases played the main role in Vietnam, both by their burden and by the attention they got from health authorities. During the last few decades, the burden of non-infectious diseases has been steadily increasing. Sometimes one speaks about the "epidemiologic transition" or "epidemiologic shift". When this concept came up in 1971 it was closely connected with a "*demographic* transition". On the one hand, many non-infectious diseases appear above all in older subjects, and on the other hand, progress in public health, medicine and rising living standards imply a higher life expectancy. These two phenomena together are leading to a higher frequency of non-infectious diseases. However, the increasing share of older people in the population is not the only factor that contributes to the rapidly growing importance of cardio-vascular diseases, cancer, diabetes and others. Factors of life-style and of the environment act as well; see e.g. Lessons 22, 23 and 25.

In this book we have treated infectious diseases before the lessons on general epidemiologic methods (Lessons 11–17 and 20, 21) but non-infectious diseases after them. As said in the Foreword the reason is in part didactic but this ordering also reflects a fundamental difference between prevention strategies for the two types of diseases. We shall expound this in Sect. 2.3.

Let us now look at the concept of a "factor" in a more systematic way.

1.3 Modern Epidemiology

The fundamental idea of modern epidemiology is to admit other "factors" in addition to the classical factors age, sex, time, place and occupation. One of the best-known factors is *smoking.* It influences frequencies of many diseases like lung cancer. In a qualitative way this simply means that lung cancer is more frequent among smokers than among non-smokers. Such factors are not routinely recorded in registers like the one of the consultations in a Commune Health Station. Hence their influence is the subject of *epidemiologic studies*. They will be the theme of a large part of the present book.

The concept of a "factor" is the core of epidemiology. This is reflected in the formal definition:

Epidemiology is the science of the distribution of diseases and other health-related features in human populations and of the factors that influence this distribution.

Whenever we attack a concrete epidemiologic problem, we have to recall this definition and give a precise and specific meaning to the words that appear in it. The rest of the present lesson will be devoted to a first discussion of these terms.

The definition refers to "human populations". They are the *target populations* already mentioned in the preceding section. For example, which target population do we have in mind when speaking about consultations in a Commune Health Station? It clearly does not consist of *all* inhabitants of the commune. It is true that basically we are interested in disease frequencies in the whole commune but some sick persons may have stayed at home or may only have consulted a private physician who does not file any reports at all. Thus from the Register of Consultations alone we cannot obtain disease frequencies in the entire commune. This trivial fact is sometimes called the "iceberg phenomenon". A more practical definition of the target population in the present situation may be to let it consist of all people who came to the station for a consultation at least once during the year in question.

In any such situation, we need to observe the following *golden rule*:

In every epidemiologic problem or statement, describe first the target population in precise terms.

1.4   Outcome Variables

The definition of epidemiology mentions "diseases and other health-related features". Let us look at the example "diastolic blood pressure". It is an individual feature in the sense that every member of the target population has, at a given moment, his or her own individual diastolic blood pressure. Another example would be the disease "influenza"; in a given month, some members of the target population did contract influenza but others did not. Often, especially in primary health facilities where diagnostic facilities are lacking, one records a *clinical* diagnosis or syndrome only, for example an "influenza syndrome". Again, this is diagnosed in some individuals of the target population and not in others. Here are three more examples: feeling depressed; having been injured; having died in the year 2016 from lung cancer.

In order to simplify the language and not to be overly pedantic, we shall in the sequel employ the term "disease" even when we are dealing with impaired health in general.

A disease at a given moment is something that depends on the individual member of the target population. It has a specific "value" for each of them. For example if Nhung suffers today from measles but Loan does not, the disease has the value "sick" for Nhung and "not sick" for Loan. It is therefore what is commonly being called a "variable".

A "variable" attributes a specific "value" to each member of the target population.

These values are of very different nature as in the examples above: blood pressure, diagnosis, feeling depressed or not, having been injured or not, having died in 2017 or not. Often one uses "coding" in order to describe them not only in words but also by numbers.

In the definition of epidemiology, we regard a disease as the *result* or the *outcome* of the influence of certain factors; hence, we call it an "*outcome* variable". A shorter term is "health outcome".

1.5   Factors (Determinants, Exposure Variables)

Like the outcome variables, the *factors* that we have in mind in the definition of epidemiology are *variables*. This means that they take a particular *value* for each individual member of the target population, which in general *varies* between members. We have already mentioned the "classical" factors age, sex, time, place and occupation. For example, in the register of consultations of a Commune Health Station, each person has *his* or *her* particular age, sex, date of consultation and address.

Modern epidemiology investigates many other factors. The factor "smoking" had already been mentioned. We might put it into the category "habits" or "life style". However, since nicotine addiction is, like any other drug addiction, a disease, we can also regard it as a "disease acting as a factor that influences another disease". There are many more examples in that category, old and new ones. Thus, a viral bronchitis favours the appearance of "opportunistic infections" such as pneumonia, AIDS has an influence on tuberculosis, a papillomavirus infection may cause cervix cancer etc.

In addition to the afore-mentioned classical factors, we can list the following categories:

- Genetic factors, or "predisposition" in a more old-fashioned terminology. For example, it has been observed for a long time already that some people are more susceptible to contract leprosy than others.
- Environmental factors, for example general hygiene, air pollution, chemicals in the house, water, soil etc. Infective agents like virus and bacteria are also included here.
- Life style factors such as personal hygiene, nutrition, smoking, sleep, stress, physical exercise and others.
- Social and economic conditions, for example education, wealth and income, housing and social standing.
- Iatrogenic factors, that is the results of the action of a physician (*"iatros"* in ancient Greek) or of any other part of the health system. Unintended consequences of a treatment, especially harmful side effects and infections in a hospital (nosocomial infections, from *"nosocomion"*, hospital, in ancient Greek) are prominent examples. We shall see in Sect. 2.2 that even the normal clinical activities "diagnosis" and "treatment" can be regarded as "factors" and studied from an epidemiologic point of view.

Epidemiologists often use the word "determinant" instead of the colourless "factor" in order to underline that they are interested in the influence of factors, which *determine* the distribution of target diseases. "Exposure variable" is another name of the same thing.

A factor can have a *benign* influence on the target disease. For example, a *treatment* of the disease, which is administered to patients with the purpose of curing the ailment, often has indeed a positive influence. If, however, we are suspecting a factor to have a *detrimental* influence and if we are investigating it under that angle, we call it a *risk* factor.

Particular subfields of the field of epidemiology may be defined by the type of variables that are involved. There are "outcome-oriented" topics such as those in the Lessons 6–10, 18, 22 and 23 and "exposure-oriented" topics like those investigated in Lessons 4, 5, 25 and 26. In the first case, one looks at a particular disease and searches for its risk factors. In the second case, one investigates outcomes of given particular exposures.

1.6 Distributions and Statistics

In the definition of epidemiology, there also appears the word "distribution". This is the technical term to which we had already alluded in the beginning of Sect. 1.2.

The distribution of a disease is given by its *frequency* in various parts of the target population.

For example, in order to describe the distribution of lung cancer in Vietnam in the year 2017 in the target population "all inhabitants of Vietnam" we can indicate its frequency in every district. The frequency in every province would provide only a less detailed description.

As said before we need to make precise what we mean by "frequency". There are two ways to do this. The frequency of a disease may be either the number of *new* cases that declare themselves during a given period of time (*incidence*) or the number of cases that *exist* at a given moment (*prevalence*). Thus the incidence of lung cancer in the province of Thaí Bình in the year 2017 is the number of cases that were newly diagnosed in Thaí Bình during that year. Its prevalence on the first January 2018 is the number of cases that existed on that date. A death frequency, also called "mortality", is of course an incidence, namely the number of deaths during a certain period.

Likewise, the *parts* or *subgroups* of the target population that appear in the definition of a distribution must be clearly defined. They normally depend on the problem with which we are dealing. For example, in classical descriptive epidemiology, they may be age groups, or the female and male part of the population, or geographic areas such as communes, districts, provinces, regions and countries or even (requiring perhaps a bit more abstract thinking) the same population regarded at different moments. In any case, the concept of a distribution is a purely statistical one.

Next, let us pass to the interpretation of the last term in the definition of epidemiology, namely "influence". We have already met many examples. By saying that the factor "age" influences the distribution of measles we mean that the incidence of measles is not the same in all age groups; measles are "age-dependent". Similarly, diarrhoea and the influenza syndrome are "time-dependent", that is, influenced by the factor "time". In particular, their incidence is not the same in all months of the year; there is a seasonal effect. The meaning of the statement "smoking influences lung cancer" is that its incidence in the two parts of the population "smokers" and "non-smokers" is different (*very* different indeed!)

Thus the concept of an *influence* in the sense of the definition of epidemiology is, again, a purely statistical one. When we study this influence in a concrete situation in precise quantitative terms, we use statistical methods. Depending on the problem these methods may be quite elementary or extremely complex and sophisticated, but the underlying idea is always the same: it is the idea of *comparing* disease frequencies between groups with different levels of the factors, i.e. of the exposure variables. For example, we compare incidences of measles in different age groups, or the incidence of diarrhoea or of the influenza syndrome in different months, or the incidence of lung cancer between smokers and non-smokers. Thus in short:

Epidemiology is a statistical subject. Its quintessence is the comparison of disease or death frequencies in groups that distinguish from each other by different values of the exposure variables.

From the early times of Public Health on, starting millennia ago, physicians and health administrators have been thinking in terms of *causes* of diseases. We have also done this already in a vague fashion when we stated that "a papillomavirus infection may cause cervix cancer". The relation between on the one hand the statistical relations studied in epidemiology and on the other hand the "aetiology", that is, the science of the causes of diseases (Greek "*aetia*", cause), is clearly a basic issue. It is, however, difficult theoretically and has been the subject of many heated discussions. We shall come back to it later in various places.

1.7 Outlook

The preceding presentation has necessarily still been fairly vague. In the following lessons the reader will first treat particular situations and problems and thus familiarize herself or himself further with the basic ideas, concepts and methods. After that, Lesson 15 will provide a more solid basis. Armed with these tools, the reader will then attack some more advanced topics.

As said in the Preface the reader should keep in mind that the purpose of the present book is to convey three things: clear *ideas* about the place of epidemiology in Public Health; its basic *concepts;* and the general principles of its *methods.* After having studied the book, she or he should be able to analyze a concrete situation in terms of these ideas, concepts and methods, to recognize the type of problem at hand and to understand what is going on. However, it is *not* intended to teach statistical *techniques* except the simplest ones. The study of an epidemiologic problem of any degree of complexity requires *teamwork* from the very beginning. In addition to a person who commands solid understanding of epidemiologic issues, indispensable for planning the study, there may also be members of the team that come from other disciplines, for example physicians, depending on the situation. Some people think that the use of statistical computer software is sufficient to handle many epidemiologic problems, but it can never replace a good comprehension of both the underlying ideas and of the principles of the statistical methods.

1.8   Practical Work

1. Visit a Commune Health Station and establish its health spectrum exclusively on the basis of the Register of Consultations, in other words without using the reports already made by the staff. Afterwards, compare both your method of calculation and your results with those used and obtained by the person that is responsible for the reports of the station. Define the target population and the outcome variables in precise terms. Analyse the influence of the factors "age", "sex" and "time" on some important diseases including injuries.
2. Find out where and how frequencies of deaths are being established in your commune.
3. Obtain from your Province Health Department or from a Central Hospital in your province the following indicators, analogous to those mentioned in Table 1.1: Mortality by causes in your province during a recent year for children under 1 year of age, and the same for children under 5. Comment on the results.

Lesson 2
Uses and Applications of Epidemiology

This lesson is a *survey* on the role of epidemiology in Public Health. The reader should not try to memorize it, but come back to it once in a while later when studying more specific lessons.

2.1 Structure of the Health System

We have recognized that epidemiology is a *subfield* of Public Health; the basic theme is always a population. It is, however, not only a subfield; it is more:

Epidemiology is the *core* of Public Health. It intervenes almost everywhere. It is the main guide in shaping the structure of a health system and in determining its activities.

In the present section, we shall sketch the role of epidemiology in shaping the *structure* of the health system. In the following sections of this lesson we shall describe how epidemiology determines the main *activities* of the health system, namely curing diseases, preventing diseases, finding cases of diseases early by screening, and defining health strategies. Details will be treated and many examples will be given in later lessons.

The *structure of health systems* in general is not our subject but in order to place the role of epidemiology in Public Health into the right perspective, we shall first outline very briefly the structure of the Vietnamese public health system, preceded by a few historical remarks on the evolution of Public Health in the world.

In ancient Rome there existed during some periods a system of public physicians appointed by municipal councillors. In China, public isolation wards for people having attracted certain infectious diseases are frequently mentioned from the Yin-Sang dynasty on (around 1350 B.C.). Later, in several countries, public authorities established clinics and hospitals as a service to the community. Public preventive health measures started essentially in the nineteenth century. They consisted mainly in advocating personal hygiene and in furthering public hygiene such as better water supply, sewage, waste disposal, and in systematic vaccinations.

© Springer Nature Switzerland AG 2019
K. Krickeberg et al., *Epidemiology*, Statistics for Biology and Health,
https://doi.org/10.1007/978-3-030-16368-6_2

In Vietnam, during the French colonial administration, small "*dispensaires*" could be found in many districts. A few large public hospitals were established. After having gained its independence, Vietnam built an all-embracing network of Commune Health Stations, policlinics, and hospitals on all levels. There are also specialized health care networks meant to deal with particular problems such as tuberculosis, malaria, and leprosy. Parallel to them, there exists a network of institutions devoted to the *prevention* of infectious diseases, in particular *hygiene*. They all come together on the commune level. Finally, there are the administrative units "District Health Centres" and "Province Health Departments", which are also concerned with finances and budgets. Several "Health Information Systems" are to insure the coherence of all of these institutions.

Present day Public Health has many facets, which are reflected in various courses of the curricula in Medical Faculties and Universities and the Hanoi University of Public Health. The main topics are, in addition to Epidemiology: Demography; Health Systems; Health Administration; Health Management; Health Economics; Health Information; Health Education and Promotion; Health Law. It is almost obvious that all of them are making use of epidemiology and could not function without it. Indeed, in order to establish and organize health stations, policlinics, and hospitals, to fix the number and type of their personnel, to build specialized health institutions like a network devoted to tuberculosis, malaria or AIDS, and to estimate the necessary financial means, we have to know the importance of the diseases to be dealt with as expressed by their frequencies, which means disease spectra and descriptive epidemiology. The first question has always been: what is needed to treat so and so many cases of such and such disease? For example, the number of beds to be foreseen in a hospital depends on the number of expected cases of diseases that require hospitalization, a trivial fact that is, however, not always sufficiently taken into account. The gravity of diseases including sequels and their importance for society measured in various ways such as lost years of life or economic losses have also been playing a role.

Likewise, in order to plan institutions devoted to hygiene, it must be known which hygienic risk factors have a detrimental influence on which diseases, for example poor water supply on cholera.

2.2 Curing Diseases

Curing diseases is the main activity of health systems all over the world, and most financial means and the overwhelming part of health personnel are devoted to it. Preventive measures are still widely neglected although in the long run they could be much more beneficial to health.

Curing diseases is generally looked upon as an activity directed at individual patients. We shall see below that it is related to Public Health indirectly through the structure of the health system. However, there also exist a few curative activities that enter the realm of Public Health directly. They are organized for a specific target population following the same rules for every patient. Under these rules, the same treatment is administered in every case according to the same fixed decision scheme that is not decided upon individually by the physician. Some special programmes such as the former "Control of Diarrhoeal Diseases (CDD)" and "Acute Respiratory Infections (ARI)" fall into this category. They are sketched in Sect. 2.5 where we shall also see that they are largely based on epidemiologic knowledge.

Let us now go back to the usual individual treatment of diseases, that is, *clinical medicine*. From a superficial point of view, it has nothing to do with epidemiology. However, how does a physician who has questioned and examined a patient establish his *diagnosis*? He believes in the diagnosis he made because he has learned in the university, from the literature, from his own experiences or from advice by colleagues that this diagnosis will be right in many, and perhaps in most cases where the anamnesis and the results of examinations were very similar to those in his particular case at hand. We shall regard the set of these "similar" cases as our target population. In this way we have already adopted the point of view of epidemiology. The diagnosis made is the input factor defined on the target population. The outcome variable takes the value "the diagnosis was correct" or "it was incorrect"; they are certainly "health-related features". This point of view may seem fairly abstract but it is in fact eminently practical.

Diagnostic rules and procedures are indeed rarely perfect. Not only in primary health care where a diagnosis is often only based on the anamnesis and clinical symptoms, but also in higher-level health care, even an excellent diagnostic procedure will usually give a wrong result for a few, and sometimes for many, cases. The desirable characteristics of a diagnostic procedure cannot be described by its performance in individual cases. They are represented by the distribution of the outcome variable defined above, for example by the proportion of correct diagnoses among all cases. In Public Health, the knowledge of these characteristics is indispensable when deciding about the purchase of diagnostic equipment or when recommending diagnostic procedures to be used. This topic belongs to *Clinical Epidemiology*; see Sect. 19.2.

The next step in case management is *treatment*. Again, the physician applies a specific treatment by relying on experiences that others or he himself have made. These experiences concern a population of cases. Evaluating the efficacy of a treatment means studying the influence of the factor "treatment" on outcomes of the type "recovery, improvement, pain relief, longer survival etc." It is an epidemiologic problem. Such an evaluation is called a *clinical trial*; see Lesson 18.

Unfortunately, many medical treatments that were or still are being taught in universities and routinely applied by physicians are based on beliefs, or on experiences that were never analyzed rigorously, and often on fashions. Quite a few have turned out to be useless or even harmful when subjected to a rigorous study. Clinical trials are meant to evaluate the performance of a treatment in a given population. It is the duty of public health authorities to see to it that only treatments are being used for which there is *evidence*, based on correct trials, of their efficacy. Clinical trials also allow us to *compare* the merits of several treatments of the same disease. All of this holds for the so-called Eastern Medicine as well as for Western Medicine; it also holds for traditional and so-called "alternative" medicine as well as for modern "school" medicine. In this respect, there ought to be no difference between them.

Clinical trials, too, are usually being considered to belong to clinical epidemiology although we shall treat them separately in Lesson 18 because of their special importance. More generally:

Clinical epidemiology is the epidemiologic, statistical evaluation of case management procedures and related activities and its application in daily clinical practice.

2.3   Preventing Diseases

When being asked "what is the most important application of epidemiology" most people working in the health sector will probably reply *"it is the prevention of diseases"*. We start with the familiar concept of prevention, which means measures to prevent the appearance of diseases (primary prevention). We shall define so-called secondary and primary prevention at the end of this section.

Preventive measures consist in reducing the level of risk factors. They rely heavily on epidemiologic knowledge.

Prevention may be an act of clinical medicine, applied to a particular person. Then it consists mostly in administering to this person a "prophylactic drug". For example somebody who intends to travel to a region infested with malaria infected Anopheles may receive from his physician a suitable drug that is both curative and preventive. Also, prophylactic drugs are sometimes given against side effects of a treatment. We shall not pursue this clinical kind of prevention.

In this book we shall deal with preventive measures applied to populations. Let us look at some examples and start with the prevention of infectious diseases. There, *immunizations* have been important and successful preventive measures. Like all preventive measures in Public Health they need to be evaluated by trials analogously to clinical trials of curative treatments. In particular, for a given vaccination procedure, we need to know its "efficacy". Vaguely speaking this is the proportion of people protected by the vaccination among those who would have fallen ill if there had been no vaccination. We also need to know the duration of this protection. The vaccination against smallpox by a vaccine obtained from cows that suffered from the "cowpox" (hence the word "vaccine" from the Latin *"vacca"*, the cow) had a particularly high and long-lasting efficacy. This allowed the eradication of the disease. Another very useful vaccination, although of slightly lower efficacy, is the one against measles. All of this will be taken up again in Sect. 5.3.

The decision whether to apply a given immunization systematically to such and such target population also depends on other types of epidemiologic knowledge. Firstly, the "weight" of the disease without such an intervention plays a role, expressed for example by its frequency, by a DALY or by the costs caused by the disease in the population in question. Secondly, there are the expected costs of the intervention. In other words one may ask oneself whether it is worthwhile to vaccinate.

It will often be advisable to restrict the measure to what is called a "high-risk group". Thirdly, there may be more efficient alternative measures. Fourth, the vaccination may cause harmful side effects to part of the population. For further discussion in concrete settings see Sects. 6.3 and 22.4.

We have already noted in the preceding Section that *classical* hygiene has a long history which can be summarized by the Public Health measures *clean water supply, sewage, waste disposal,* and *education for cleanliness*. These have been the main measures to prevent infectious diseases, a long time before immunizations. For example, knowing that cholera is predominantly spread by water polluted by faeces, its control rests on providing unpolluted water. In the early twentieth century tuberculosis diminished much in many countries because of higher hygienic standards.

Some infectious diseases are being controlled by direct interventions, too, like destroying the vectors of the infective agent in the case of malaria or dengue fever; see Sects. 4.6, 7.2 and 8.4. Lessons 6–10 will provide more information on specific infectious diseases.

Let us now pass to the prevention of *non-infectious* diseases. The main ones, namely cardiovascular diseases, cancer and diabetes mellitus, are a steadily increasing burden on the population. All the possible risk factors categorized in Sect. 1.5 play a role. Their list as established by epidemiologic studies is getting longer all the time, but their knowledge also provides more and more possibilities for prevention. Smoking is now already a classical example but unfortunately still very actual. In order to reduce the incidence of lung cancer and numerous other health defects, Public Health measures are required to reduce smoking. Smoking is an addiction and people usually start smoking because of social pressure; in that sense one might even say that smoking is a *contagious* disease. Hence Public Health measures need to focus in the first place on keeping people, especially the young ones, from *starting* to smoke. Appropriate measures are the complete prohibition of direct and indirect publicity for cigarettes, making it very hard to buy them, taxing them heavily, forbidding to smoke in public places, and an *intelligent* wide-spread health education directed especially at the youth.

Many more examples from each of the categories of factors listed in Sect. 1.5 will be given in Lessons 22, 23, 25 and 26.

For infectious diseases, there is also the indirect *preventive* effect of *curative* treatments, which is an analogue to the indirect effect of vaccinations mentioned in Sect. 1.1. Let us look at a fairly recent example, namely drug treatment of AIDS; see Sect. 10.5. By treating a large part of the patients at an early stage, the number of persons carrying the virus who can infect others will be significantly reduced, which will result in a lower incidence. Thus the curative treatment becomes a preventive act as well. More generally:

A fundamental difference between the epidemiology of infectious and of non-infectious diseases consists in the fact that the incidence of the former can be influenced by curative treatments of diseased persons (indirect effect) but the incidence of the latter cannot.

Indeed, if somebody would find a treatment that would cure all lung cancers and if this treatment would be applied systematically as a Public Health measure, the incidence of lung cancer would not decrease. It might even increase because more people, knowing of the treatment, would no longer be deterred from smoking.

We shall therefore include a section on case management in several lessons dealing with particular infectious diseases but not in lessons about non-infectious diseases. Indirect effects are being studied theoretically by mathematical models; see Sect. 5.2 for the general idea of modelling the evolution of an infectious disease in a population.

When discussing the prevention of non-infectious diseases we did it in terms of risk factors: prevention means reducing the level of known *risk factors.* From a more formal point of view this holds as well for infectious diseases. Indeed when for example planning, executing and following-up a vaccination campaign in a well-defined population the underlying risk factor is "absence of vaccination". Absence of hygiene can also be looked upon as a risk factor. This point of view may be regarded as far-fetched and abstract but it is, like the analogous conception of diagnosis in Sect. 1.2, quite practical. It turns out that the "efficacy"of a vaccination is nothing else but a particular case of a basic general concept of epidemiology called the "etiological fraction among the exposed"; see Sect. 15.1. This allows in particular to use software developed for epidemiologic studies of risks also in the evaluation of vaccinations.

Nowadays the term "hygiene" is often being used in the broader sense of fighting the risk factors for any ailments, not only for infectious diseases. One talks for example about "mental hygiene".

Prevention in the sense of the present section means lowering the incidence of a disease. It is sometimes called "primary prevention". In contrast, one denotes by "secondary prevention" measures that apply to cases which have already started; these measures are early detection and early treatment. Early successful treatment shortens the average duration of the disease and thereby reduces its prevalence; see Sect. 15.1. We may for example think of tuberculosis. Secondary prevention is essentially identical with screening as treated in the following section.

There is also the concept of "tertiary prevention", which covers long-term measures for reducing invalidating effects of the disease and restoring health. It coincides largely with what is called "rehabilitation".

In this book, "prevention" will always mean "primary prevention" unless noted otherwise.

2.4 Screening

Screening means examining all members of a population in order to detect cases of the "target disease" at an early stage when they have not yet given rise to symptoms that might motivate the patient to consult a physician.

The purpose is mainly to treat the cases detected at a moment when the chances of curing them are still high. For infectious diseases screening may also serve to isolate sources of infection. It will be treated in Sect. 19.3; let us give here a brief overview.

One of the earliest target diseases of screening as an organized activity of Public Health was tuberculosis. In many countries, screening was done in schools by the Mendel-Mantoux-test. School doctors also performed screening for other diseases, for example dental caries, which is, as we now know, essentially a disease caused by bacteria. In Vietnam there exist in addition screening programmes in schools for trachoma, disorders of eye refraction, impaired hearing, malnutrition, and perhaps other ailments. Cases are sent to the relevant medical service for treatment.

At the present time, various forms of cancer are prominent target diseases for screening. Examples are cancer of the female breast, cervix cancer, colon cancer, and prostate cancer; see Sect. 22.4. Screening for lung cancer still presents serious problems.

Epidemiologic knowledge intervenes in screening programmes in two ways. Firstly, it is needed in order to determine the appropriate population to be screened. As for almost any other Public Health measure, the advantages of screening in a concrete situation need to be weighed against its cost and possible side effects. Hence one would normally restrict it to *high-risk* groups, that is, to populations where the frequency and burden of the target disease is relatively high. Screening for *occupational* diseases is an obvious example.

Secondly, epidemiology intervenes in screening programmes in the form of *clinical epidemiology*. In order to plan and evaluate such a programme, the characteristics of the diagnostic procedure to be used must be known. Loosely speaking, we must know which proportion of the existing cases can be detected correctly by our diagnostic "test". Often, there are several possible tests to chose from, for example for pulmonary tuberculosis there is the X-ray examination and a sputum analysis. The choice will depend on their epidemiologic characteristics in addition to cost and side effects.

2.5 Health Strategies

Many curative and preventive activities of the health system go on in a fairly routine manner. Their framework and their content change only slowly as time passes. Sometimes, however, new problems require special strategies. New approaches may also be needed to old problems that have become particularly big and urgent. *Emerging diseases* such as AIDS cause new problems. Most of these diseases are infectious but not all. In Vietnam, *obesity* is a slowly, and *injuries by traffic accidents* a rapidly emerging non-infectious health problem. Tuberculosis, cardiovascular diseases, most forms of cancer, chronic respiratory diseases, diabetes mellitus, and musculoskeletal disorders are old problems of increasing importance.

The planning of a health strategy to handle a specific problem must take many features into account, in particular economic, administrative, and social ones in addition to epidemiologic elements. In this section, we restrict ourselves to mentioning the role of such epidemiologic elements in a few typical examples; more detailed descriptions will be given in later lessons.

Tuberculosis and malaria institutes and networks were established in Vietnam in the early 1960s. They had to define their strategy at the beginning and to adapt it later to changing epidemiologic conditions. There are several similarities in the way the two strategies operate. This is due to the fact that both target diseases are mainly *chronic* infections that require a follow-up of patients. Both networks pursue curative *and* preventive work.

The public health programmes CDD (Control of Diarrhoeal Diseases) and ARI (Acute Respiratory Infections) were, on the contrary, concerned with *acute* infections to be treated normally in a single consultation. They were essentially *curative.* The basic idea of CDD was to cure a dehydration due to diarrhoea by oral rehydration, and ARI consisted in rapid diagnosis of bacterial acute respiratory infections, especially pneumonia, and treatment by antibiotics. Their epidemiologic foundation is again two fold: monitoring the incidence of the target diseases including mortality due to them, and knowing the characteristics of the diagnostic and curative procedures. Both programmes are now integrated into the routine activities of the public health system.

CDD is an example of a simple, cheap and efficient strategy, which was, however, implemented only a long time after its epidemiologic foundation had been laid. The efficacy of oral rehydration was in fact already studied in the late 1930s but CDD was implemented in Vietnam in the early 1980s.

Avian influenza is a recently emerging disease. No reasonable strategy has been generally accepted. Would it consist in stocking vast amounts of an antiviral drug? In a mass vaccination of poultry? In vaccinating human populations? In a combination of these measures? In destroying suspected herds of poultry? In other measures to break the chain of transmission to be described in Sect. 4.6? The decision would depend, in addition to cost and organization, on the efficacy of each of these measures and on another epidemiologic element, namely the dynamics of the transmission of the infection; see again Lesson 5.

Adding fluoride to toothpaste has been a successful strategy to prevent dental caries whereas fluoridation of drinking water is controversial. Definitive epidemiologic investigations are still wanting.

The health authorities of many countries have designed special strategies for preventing cancer or cardio-vascular diseases; see Sects. 22.4 and 23.3.

2.6 Practical Work

1. Visit a District Health Centre and inquire about the budget for the various health activities of the district. Look at the details and try to find out to which extent the allocation of funds is being determined by epidemiologic aspects.

2. Describe the activities called "Mother and Child Health" (MCH) in terms of the concepts of the present lesson: Place of the care (to be visited); organization (by whom; special programme or not); type of activities (curative, preventive, screening); epidemiologic bases.
3. Inform yourself about screening for occupational diseases in a selected industrial or agricultural enterprise in one of the provinces you know. Visit an enterprise where some occupations are considered "dangerous", for example a larger pottery where fumes from paints may be noxious.

Lesson 3
Some Case Studies and Situation Analyses

Before presenting basic ideas of epidemiology in a systematic way, we look at some typical epidemiologic settings that provide a first insight.

3.1 Traffic Accidents

We have said in Sect. 1.1 that in the twentieth century the term "epidemiology" took a much wider meaning than before when it concerned only infectious diseases. This semantic transition reflected a transition of the "disease spectrum"; non-infectious ailments and injuries played now an increasing role. In Vietnam, we may indeed very well speak of "epidemics" of, among others, cancer, cardio-vascular diseases, type 2 diabetes, and injuries by crashes in road traffic. Hence, we shall start the present lesson by describing a study about the descriptive epidemiology of traffic accidents.

This study was conducted in the city of Thaí Bình in the framework of a joint project called SAVE of Vietnamese, German, and Hungarian Medical Universities, which also comprised a clinical part regarding trauma and emergency medicine, and road safety programmes in schools. It began by a literature search and informal observations in order to identify the main issues to be investigated further in a rigorous way. They turned out to look like this:

- Injuries and deaths by road traffic crashes have significantly increased in Vietnam from 1994 to 2002.
- Official sources document only about 22–60% of all non-fatal injuries.
- Crashes in road traffic affect young and middle-income persons much more than in proportion to their share of the population.
- In rural communities, riding a two-wheel vehicle, that is a bicycle or motorcycle, is the leading source of injuries.
- Wearing a helmet reduces the risk of head injuries.
- Only about one third of all motorcyclists wear a helmet.

© Springer Nature Switzerland AG 2019
K. Krickeberg et al., *Epidemiology*, Statistics for Biology and Health,
https://doi.org/10.1007/978-3-030-16368-6_3

Next, a study was planned. The population to be studied consisted of all students in two colleges in Thaí Bình City; they are indeed young and mainly middle class road users. This is what we shall call the "target population". From the target population, a sample of 1000 students was drawn by a random mechanism. They were given fairly elaborate questionnaires, which were correctly filled in and returned by 662 students. These 662 people will henceforth be referred to as the "subjects in the study" or the "study population" or "study sample".

The statistical evaluation of their answers in the questionnaires gave the following results. First, there was a purely descriptive part where by "Percentage" we mean "Percentage of subjects in the sample":

- Mean age: 22 years.
- Male-female ratio: 0.76:1.
- Percentage riding regularly a motorcycle: 35.5%.
- Percentage driving another motorized vehicle: 1.2%.
- Percentage riding a bicycle: 55.1%.
- Percentage using the road only as pedestrians: 8.2%.
- Percentage already involved in a road traffic crash: 22%.

Restricting ourselves now to the motorized individuals in the sample (36.7% of the whole sample) and indicating percentages among these only, we describe their "risky" habits:

- Using a motorcycle to transport heavy goods: 36%.
- Using a mobile phone while driving or riding: 23%.
- Driving or riding under the influence of alcohol: 16%.
- Not holding a valid driver's license: 7%.
- Not always following traffic rules: 7%.
- Like to drive fast: 26%.

Among motorcyclists (35.5% of the whole sample), 82% own a helmet but only 48% always wear it when it is required.

Regarding sources of information about road safety for the whole sample, the following percentages came out: Television 74%; school or college 47%; friends 27%; newspapers 26%; radio 26%; family 24%. Motorized road users are more likely than non-motorized ones to select a particular source in the questionnaire.

Next the study was analyzed in the sense of the basic idea of epidemiology as sketched in Sect. 1.3, that is the influence of risk factors. Among subjects in the study population the "outcome" to be investigated was a road traffic crash in which the subject was involved and which she or he remembered and reported. The result:

It turned out that the following factors "significantly" raised the frequency of crashes as remembered by the subjects:

- Driving under the influence of alcohol.
- Using a mobile phone while driving.
- Transporting heavy goods.

An influence of the following factors on the frequency of remembered crashes could not be proved:

- Gender.
- Age.
- Type of road use.
- Knowledge of traffic rules.
- Holding a valid driver's license.
- For motorcyclists: wearing a helmet.
- Enjoy driving or riding fast.

The question arises of course what we mean by "significantly" or "could not be proved". For example, if the frequency of crashes were just *a little bit* lower among women than among men, we would be inclined to say that an influence of the factor "gender" could not be proved. If on the contrary it were *much* lower, we would consider this as significant evidence of an influence of the factor. Where is the borderline between "a little bit" and "much"? Statistical questions of this kind will be treated in later lessons, in particular in Sects. 14.3 and 14.4.

The concept of "frequency" also needs to be made precise.

There is one more important methodological issue. If, for example, we want to analyze the influence of the factor "Enjoy driving or riding fast" on the occurrence of crashes, we could naïvely think of two alternative approaches:

- Compare the frequency of remembered crashes among those who enjoy going fast with the analogous frequency among those who do not enjoy going fast.
- Compare the frequency of subjects who enjoy going fast among those who remember a crash with the analogous frequency among those who do not remember a crash.

These are quite different methods. The question of which one is legitimate in the present setting will also be taken up later, especially in Sect. 20.2.

Technically speaking, this study is "cross-sectional", which means that we use a single sample at a given moment and utilize the information available at that moment. We shall treat this concept more in detail in Lesson 16.

Finally, what is the ultimate goal of such studies? The legal framework for the prevention of injuries and deaths by traffic accidents exists in Vietnam. There are the mandatory helmet law, general traffic laws, and new law enforcement rules. Hence the main contribution to road safety should now come from educational campaigns. Studies like the present one are indispensable for designing efficient campaigns. Indeed, knowing the risk factors in a quantitative way permits to optimize the content of messages. Knowing the sources of information quoted by motorcyclist permits to utilize those sources that promise to be particularly helpful in education about safe riding.

3.2 A Cholera Outbreak

Investigating and controlling an outbreak of an infectious disease is a classical task of public health. The first questions to be asked are: what was the source of the outbreak, which factors have contributed to it, and along which paths did the infection travel? Answering these questions is indispensable for answering the following one: how can we control, contain and perhaps eliminate the epidemic that was about to break out? The outbreak of cholera in Northern Vietnam in 2007–2008 will serve us as an example. The following short report is based on training material of WHO on "field epidemiology".

On 23rd October 2007, a physician at the hospital Bach Mai in Hanoi saw a case of acute severe watery diarrhoea. The patient was a 73 year-old rice farmer. The analysis of a stool sample by the National Institute of Hygiene and Epidemiology (NIHE) was available on the morning of the next day. It showed that the man was infected by *Vibrio cholerae* of the serogroup 01, biotype El Tor, serotype Ogawa. Provincial health authorities were alerted and an "epidemic response team" formed that included an epidemiologist from NIHE, a microbiologist, and a specialist in food safety. The team conducted an outbreak investigation in the patient's village by doing the following:

- It interviewed his family and inquired in particular about food consumed during the 5 days before he fell ill.
- It took samples of water in and around his house from containers, drainpipes, and toilets.
- It collected stool samples from his household contacts.
- It asked staff of the Commune Health Station to look for other cases of acute watery diarrhoea.

As a result of this investigation and of the anamnesis at Bach Mai the following facts were established:

- The patient had attended a wedding ceremony on the 21st October and a funeral on the 23rd but had not travelled otherwise.
- No other guests at these two events became ill with acute watery diarrhoea.
- At the wedding, the man had eaten beef, chicken, and duck and drunken beer; at the funeral he had duck and water.
- On the 22nd, he had consumed dog meat and beer.

On the 26th another man, from the Hoang Mai district of Hanoi, was diagnosed at Bach Mai as suffering from acute severe watery diarrhoea. His case was handled similarly. It was found that:

- During the last 2 weeks the man had not travelled and not attended any gatherings.
- No one else in his family became ill.
- On the 22nd the family ate dog meat with shrimp paste, herbs, and raw vegetables.
- On the 23rd the family ate shrimps, minced meat, and herbs wrapped in leaves and fried.

In both cases samples of food eaten were not available.

Then, in the following days, health facilities of Northern Vietnam saw many new cases of acute severe watery diarrhoea. Each one was investigated along the same lines, including an inquiry into food consumption in restaurants. During the year 2007, there were 976 cases. The epidemic slowed down in January and February 2008 with only 10 cases but two more waves occurred later in that year. Altogether, 3017 cases of acute severe watery diarrhoea were diagnosed among which 836 had a positive stool culture for *Vibrio cholerae* of the same type.

NIHE tried to get an overview on the outbreak as a whole and not only on single cases studied separately; this is the essence of an outbreak investigation. For each day, the number of cases that had been reported up to then was computed; this gave the so-called "epidemic curve". A spot map of cases was made. The information on patients that had been recorded was analyzed statistically. This provided in particular an insight into their food consumption. As a result, certain types of food appeared as possible sources of an infection, above all dog meat. For example, four subjects whose cases were confirmed to be cholera had eaten at the same dog meat restaurant.

But what can we conclude from these observations? After all, the rest of the population that had not suffered from cholera may have had the same nutritional habits as the cases, may have eaten just as much dog meat at the same places etc. Then the data about the consumption of dog meat by the patients alone would hardly be evidence of dog meat as a source of infection.

In order to study the role of dog meat, we have to *compare* its consumption by patients with its consumption by "non-patients", that is, people who did not fall ill.

This is the basic idea of a "case-control study" where "controls" are selected from among people who did not have watery diarrhoea; see Lesson 20. Such a study was conducted by NIHE. It confirmed that dog meat was indeed a highly probable source of infection.

In May 2009, NIHE found *Vibrio cholerae* in a few dog slaughterhouses in the Ha Dong district of Ha Noi.

It was now fairly obvious which control measures were to be taken. Slaughterhouses and restaurants serving dog meat had to submit to strict hygienic controls. To interrupt a possible transmission from person to person or household to household through contaminated food or water, people living in what was considered a high-risk area were vaccinated against cholera.

3.3 Treatment of Tuberculosis and the Beijing Genotype of the Pathogen

In Vietnam as in many other countries, patients who are smear-positive for tuberculosis normally receive a standardized first-line drug treatment called "directly observed therapy, short course" (DOTS). Sometimes, it fails; then a second-line drug treatment is applied which, however, is much more expensive and has severe side effects. A main factor contributing to failure of the first-line treatment is *multidrug resistance* of the pathogen *Mycobacterium tuberculosis* to the principal drugs employed.

Several studies in the past seemed to suggest that there is an additional factor for treatment failure, namely the presence of a new "Beijing" genotype of *M. tuberculosis*. Recently epidemiologists from Vietnam and the Netherlands conducted a study in the province of Tiên Giang in order to investigate this problem further. We are going to describe the essentials.

The investigators registered data on all smear-positive patients who came to one of three selected district tuberculosis units or to the provincial tuberculosis hospital between the 1st July 2003 and the 30th June 2007. In addition to personal data, there were data on the genotype of the pathogen, drug resistance, new or previously treated patient, and treatment adherence (compliance). After exclusion of a few people for various reasons, 1106 patients remained; they formed the "study population".

The genotype of the pathogen now determined two "cohorts" of people. The first cohort consisted of all patients whose pathogen was of the Beijing genotype; it comprised 380 people. The second cohort was formed by the patients infected by a "non-Beijing" genotype; it numbered 726 people. In this context, the presence or absence of the Beijing genotype is the "exposure variable".

The investigators followed all members of the two cohorts until the result of the first-line treatment was known: either failure or success. This is the "outcome variable". It turned out that there were

- 20 failures among the 380 patients affected by the Beijing genotype (first cohort).
- 13 failures among the 726 patients affected by the "non-Beijing" genotype (second cohort).

We can use these numbers to calculate "risks" of failure. In the "Beijing cohort", this risk is equal to $20/380 = 0.053 = 5.3\%$; in the "non-Beijing cohort", it is $13/726 = 0.018 = 1.8\%$. Therefore the risk of failure is $0.053/0.018 = 2.94 \approx 3$ times higher in the first cohort than in the second one. This quotient of the risks in the two cohorts is called the "relative risk" or "risk ratio".

Thus it looks as if the presence of the Beijing genotype does indeed contribute much to treatment failure. However, what we have found is only a purely statistical association between the genotype and the result of the first-line treatment. Is there also a *causal* relation? Recall that resistance is an important factor for treatment failure. Moreover one knew that the two factors "resistance" and "genotype" are closely tied to each other; drug resistance is much higher among the Beijing genotype pathogen. The investigators therefore compared the risks of treatment failure in two cohorts where the genotype was *different* but the drug resistance *the same*. It turned out that the failure rate was also the same! Thus the difference of failure rates found above is due to a different drug resistance in the two cohorts, not to different genotypes. In modern terminology, the factor "drug resistance" is called a "confounder" of the action of the factor "genotype"; it gives rise to an apparent effect of the factor "genotype" that in reality does not exist.

To summarize:

In a cohort study, two cohorts of persons are defined by two different values of the exposure variable; one then compares the outcomes in the two cohorts with each other.

The concept of a "confounder" is fundamental in epidemiology; for details see Lesson 21.

3.4 A Clinical Trial

Benign wounds of the cervix including polyps and papillomas are fairly frequent. In order to get an idea of their prevalence in the province of Thaí Bình, an investigator chose two districts in this province, and then three communes in each of these districts. To this end, she used a "random" mechanism that was not specified further. Then she drew a sample of 400 married women in childbearing age from 18 to 49 years from these 6 communes by what is called a "systematic" sampling plan; for its definition, which is irrelevant at the present moment, see Sect. 12.2. In this sample, about 65% women suffered from one or the other type of these wounds. It was also found that their prevalence was significantly higher among women having already given birth, having had many induced abortions by scraping or suction, having a history of gynaecological infections or having married early.

There are several ways to treat benign wounds of the cervix. The objective of the present study was to compare two of them: – Galvanocautery (treatment 1); – Use of Laser CO_2 (treatment 2). First, the study population was recruited. It consisted of 102 married women aged 18–49 years who were examined between April and December 2009 in the Gynaecological Department of the University Hospital of Thaí Bình and were diagnosed as suffering from a benign wound of the cervix according to certain precise diagnostic criteria. Each patient was attributed his number of arrival, and the study population was divided into two groups as follows: group nr. 1 consisted of all women having an odd arrival number and group nr. 2 comprised those who had an even arrival number. Then all women who belonged to group nr. 1 were assigned to the treatment 1 and those in group nr. 2 got the treatment 2.

The study was evaluated by comparing the healing rate, the time to healing, and complications in the two groups. The results are given in Table 3.1. The pattern of complications was similar in both groups.

This study was a typical clinical trial of a classical type. It was a "controlled" trial because the efficacy of the Laser CO_2 treatment was evaluated by comparing it

Table 3.1 Treatment of cervic wounds

Group	1	2
Healing rate	81.6%	94.3%
Average time to healing (days)	57.6	53.7

with the efficacy of the "control" treatment by galvanocautery. It was not, however, a "randomized" trial in the modern sense because the two groups were not determined by a random mechanism. It is conceivable although not very likely that the way of constructing the two groups was not independent of the outcome of the treatments. Moreover, the trial was not "blinded". Each patient knew to which treatment she had been assigned, and the physicians who evaluated the result knew it, too. This could have influenced the judgment about healing and healing times in some cases.

Finally, why do we conduct clinical trials?

The ultimate goal of a clinical trial is to evaluate treatments in view of their use in practice in a certain population, which we call the "target population".

In our example, the target population might consist of all married Vietnamese women aged 18–49 years who are diagnosed during the coming decade in a hospital as suffering from a benign wound of the cervix. The question then arises to which extent we can draw conclusions about the efficacy of the treatments in question in such a target population if we have investigated them only in the study population of the trial. We shall deal with all of these questions in later lessons, in particular 12, 14 and 18.

Lesson 4
Infectious Diseases: Descriptive Epidemiology, Transmission, Surveillance, Control

This lesson describes some concepts and tools needed for understanding and applying the epidemiology of infectious diseases.

4.1 Definitions, History

We shall be employing the following definition of an infectious disease, which is short and focuses on the essential:

An infectious disease is a disease caused by a microorganism.

Some people use the term "communicable" as a synonym for "infectious" but there is no general agreement about its meaning. For us a communicable disease is infectious and can be transmitted directly from an infected person to another one. In everyday language the term "contagious" is preferred to "communicable".

By a microorganism we mean a living organism at the limit of visibility by the human eye or smaller. In essentially decreasing order of size, there are the following categories of microorganisms:

- Parasites and fungi.
- Bacteria including *Rickettsia, Chlamydia, Spirochaeta* and others.
- Viruses.
- Prions.

All medical students learn a lot about them in the course of their studies. Hence we shall recall here only some examples including a few historical remarks. That certain diseases are caused by invisible *living* agents was suggested in the early sixteenth century by the Italian scientist Girolamo Fracastoro, who was studying the then emerging syphilis epidemic. In the sequel, this thesis was much contested but in 1840 the German physician Jakob Henle showed that *scabies* are caused by *mites*. These parasites measure up to 0.4 mm and can therefore still be detected by the naked eye. This seems to be the first example of a confirmed infection by a living micropathogen.

© Springer Nature Switzerland AG 2019
K. Krickeberg et al., *Epidemiology*, Statistics for Biology and Health,
https://doi.org/10.1007/978-3-030-16368-6_4

In Vietnam the most important disease caused by a parasite is *malaria*. Its pathogen, a *Plasmodium*, was discovered in 1880 in Algeria by the French physician Alphonse Laveran. Other examples are *helminthiasis* and skin diseases caused by *fungi*.

The second half of the nineteenth century was above all the era of the discovery of *bacterial* pathogens (from the Greek "*bacterion*", little stick). In 1854, the Italian pathologist Filippo Pacini observed under the microscope the bacteria that cause *cholera* and attributed the disease to them. The German physician Robert Koch succeeded in 1883 in growing them in vitro. The year before, he had discovered the bacterium that gives rise to *tuberculosis*. A related bacterium is the agent of *leprosy*; its discovery in 1873 is due to the Norwegian physician Gerhard Armauer Hansen. In 1884, the German physician Friedrich Löffler found the bacterium that causes *diphtheria* and in 1906 the Belgian bacteriologist Jules Bordel discovered the bacterium leading to *pertussis*. The bacterium at the root of *tetanus* was first cultivated in vitro in 1889 by the Japanese physician Shibasaburo Kitasato who worked at that time in Berlin in the laboratory of Robert Koch. A final example in our enumeration of specific bacterial pathogens of some importance in Vietnam is that of the *plague*. It was discovered in 1894 in Hong Kong by the Swiss born French physician Alexandre Yersin. Let us recall that Yersin became one of the founding fathers of the modern Vietnamese health system. In 1895, he started building up the Pasteur Institute of Nha Trang where he lived, with short interruptions, until his death in 1943.

Bacteria play a partial role in the pathogenesis of two more diseases of great importance in Vietnam. *Acute pneumonia* is mainly due to various bacteria. *Acute diarrhoea* can be caused by parasites as well as by bacteria and by viruses.

Let us pass to viruses. The Latin word "*virus*" means both "mucus" and "poison". The Roman medical writer Aulus Cornelius Celsus used it in a medical context in the early first century when he designated sputum that transmitted *rabies* as poisonous. As it happens, rabies is indeed also a viral disease in the present sense! However, the modern investigation of viruses started in the last decade of the nineteenth century not with human but with plant and animal diseases. We shall simply list some viral infections that played or play an essential role in Vietnam: some forms of diarrhoea, AIDS, dengue fever, influenza, Japanese encephalitis, various forms of viral hepatitis, measles, poliomyelitis and smallpox.

"Prions" (proteinaceous infectious particles) may not be *living* organisms according to current definitions but this is irrelevant for the epidemiology of diseases caused by them such as the *Creutzfeld-Jacob* disease.

4.2 Infectious Diseases in the World and in Vietnam: Descriptive Epidemiology

For the whole world, we shall again restrict ourselves to looking at mortalities. From the Table 1.1 we see that in the year 2016, lower respiratory infections were the third most frequent cause of death among all causes, diarrhoeal diseases eighth and tuberculosis ninth.

Table 4.1 Incidence of, and mortality by, acute infectious diseases in Vietnam in 2007 per 100,000 inhabitants

	Dengue fever	Varicella	Shigellosis	Amoebiasis	Viral hepatitis	Typhoid	Cholera	Viral encephalitis
Incidence/ 100,000	123	43	40	16	11	3	2	1
Mortality/ 100,000	0.101	0.001	0.002	0	0.004	0.001	0	0.035

The situation of infectious diseases is now largely a more "classical" subject than that of non-infectious ones and we therefore present data about a few years back. Table 4.1 is about the eight *acute* infectious diseases of highest incidence in Vietnam in 2007. It gives rounded relative incidences and mortalities as reported to the Ministry of Health.

For *chronic* infectious diseases, prevalence is usually a more interesting indicator. For malaria, the Health Statistics Yearbook 2007 of the Vietnamese Ministry of Health gave, per 100,000 inhabitants, a prevalence of 83.27 and a mortality of 0.02. For tuberculosis in 2009 these numbers were 307 and 23, respectively as reported by the National Tuberculosis Programme; the prevalence of AFB (Acid-fast bacillus smear)-positive cases per 100,000 persons was 197. For HIV/AIDS, the prevalence of HIV-infections is the most revealing indicator. In 2007 and per 100,000 inhabitants it was roughly 340. The mortality by AIDS per 100,000 was around 20–40 depending on the sources of information. Lessons 7 and 10 contain further details, in particular about the decrease of HIV/AIDS as a cause of death since 2007.

4.3   Specific Features of the Epidemiology of Infectious Diseases

In many respects the epidemiology of infectious diseases does not differ from that of non-infectious ones. Most factors listed in Sects. 1.2 and 1.5 exert an influence on the distribution of infectious diseases as we will see later in Lessons 6–10. In this section, we shall discuss five aspects that are *specific* to the epidemiology of infectious diseases.

Firstly, the factor *infection* plays of course a special role among all other factors. Secondly, and as a consequence of this special role of the infection, there are certain risk factors such as the *lack of hygiene* that are most important in the epidemiology of infectious diseases but less so in the epidemiology of non-infectious ones. The third specific aspect is the dynamics of the *transmission* of the disease in a population, which can be modelled mathematically. There, a fourth specific feature often intervenes, namely the direct and indirect action of *immunity*, and a fifth specific trait, already described in Sect. 2.3, namely the *indirect effect* of a systematic curative strategy on prevention. Let us dwell a bit on these five features.

The factor "infection" distinguishes indeed the epidemiology of infectious diseases from that of others. The infection is *necessary* in the sense that a non-infected person cannot fall ill with the specific disease at hand. For example, if a physician has diagnosed a patient as having contracted the plague, this patient must necessarily have been infected before by *Yersinia pestis.*

This remark is not quite as obvious as it may seem at first sight because it assumes that we have a precise definition of the disease in question. In the preceding example we suppose that in his diagnosis the physician has employed the traditional description and definition of the plague by clinical symptoms. However, after the discovery of pathogens, physicians started to *define* several diseases no longer clinically but by specific pathogens, for example hepatitis B or avian influenza $A|H_5N_1$. This evolution of disease definitions can be very well observed by comparing the first International Classification of Diseases that was issued in 1893 by the International Statistical Institute under the name "International List of Causes of Death" with the tenth revision of 1994.

The factor "infection" is necessary but in general not *sufficient* for an individual to contract the disease. For example, a single *Corynebacterium diphtheriae* that manages to adhere to the wall of the pharynx of a child does normally not lead to a case of diphtheria. Likewise, a contact with a source of infection, for example with a patient suffering from influenza, is not sufficient to transmit the disease. The transmission of infectious diseases is described in *epidemiologic* terms that concern *populations*, not single individuals. They will be treated in the following lesson; a typical concept that intervenes here is the so-called "force of infection".

The second specific aspect of the epidemiology of infectious diseases, namely the special role of hygiene and similar factors, had already been mentioned briefly in Sect. 2.3. We shall come back to it in Lessons 6–10.

The third specific feature that singles out the epidemiology of infectious diseases from general epidemiology is the "dynamics" of their transmission and evolution in a given target population. It makes use of concepts such as force of infection as mentioned above. It is at the root of strategies in order to fight the disease and will be discussed in the following lesson. In this discussion, the fourth specific feature of the epidemiology of infectious diseases, namely *immunity*, will play a basic role.

The fifth trait that distinguishes infectious diseases from non-infectious ones was discussed in Sect. 2.3, namely the preventive role of curative treatments.

In the remaining part of this lesson, we shall lay the ground for the investigation of the transmission of infectious diseases. We start by looking at their path in a few typical examples.

4.4 Paths of Transmission

Whatever the path of transmission of an infectious disease may be, the pathogen enters the human body through one or several of the following ports:

- Via the *digestive* system, e.g. hepatitis A.
- Via the *respiratory* tract, e.g. influenza.

- Via the *skin* and *mucous membranes* and from there through *blood vessels* or *lymph capillaries*, e.g. hepatitis B, dengue fever, malaria, syphilis and plague.

Some diseases are transmitted more or less directly from person to person in various ways, for example influenza and tuberculosis by droplets, poliomyelitis faecally-orally and syphilis by sexual contact. They are called *contagious.* Contagion of measles can take place through the air by droplets even over some distance.

The infection may also take a longer route through a *non-living* medium. For cholera, the medium is water. For paratyphoid, the agent *Salmonella paratyphi* is mainly transmitted by foodstuff.

For many diseases, the infection passes through a *living vector.* In Vietnam the main diseases transmitted in this way are malaria and dengue fever whose vectors are, respectively, *Anopheles* and *Aedes* mosquitoes. A mosquito becomes infected when biting an infected person and then infects, in turn, another person by biting it.

Infection by the plague follows a more complicated path. In the past, the prevailing mechanism looked like this: the pathogen was transmitted by flea bites among migrating rats (*Rattus norvegicus*) and among domestic rats (*Rattus rattus*) but also between these two species. The passage from rats, mainly from domestic ones, to humans and back happened through fleas, too. This resulted in the well-known *epidemics* of the past. In recent times, the disease has become *endemic* in several countries. There are permanent *herds*, or *reservoirs*, of the disease among rodents, mainly in forests. From there, the infection gets to humans via various species of rats, always with fleas as the intermediate host of the agent.

Thus, plague in modern times has an animal reservoir of the pathogen independently of humans, which forms the *source* of the process of transmission. Leptospirosis is another example; many mammals may host bacteria of the family *Leptospiraceae.* They pass from the urine of infected animals to humans via skin lesions or mucous membranes. There is no direct transmission between humans.

4.5 Epidemic Surveillance

Both the surveillance and the control of an infectious disease obviously depend very much on the specific characteristics of the disease. The source of infection and the reservoirs, its possible paths, the force of infection and other epidemiologic parameters play a decisive role. We shall therefore illustrate essential ideas later in Lessons 6–10 by looking at particular diseases and restrict ourselves in the present lesson to a few common principles.

Modern epidemic surveillance is a vast field. The following definition has been given:

Epidemic surveillance is the collection, transfer, analysis and interpretation of information related to cases of infectious diseases, which is organized in the form of a permanent system.

Such a permanent organization excludes studies that are performed expressly in order to obtain insight into a particular problem by the methods that will be described in Lessons 15–21 and 24. The field of epidemic surveillance is also to be distinguished from that of *outbreak investigations*. The latter concern the various ways in which a particular infectious disease appears at a particular time. Surveillance often serves as a tool for the investigation of outbreaks. The main goal of both surveillance and outbreak investigation is the *control* of the infectious diseases in question.

Any surveillance starts at the *source of information*. Sometimes information on cases of an infectious disease is obtained by screening (Sects. 2.4 and 19.3). Another source is so-called *active case finding* where health workers visit households, schools, factories, homes for the elderly, prisons etc. or even health facilities in order to discover cases; in some countries this is being done for malaria. The normal source, however, is *passive* case finding in health facilities. A patient consults for example a Commune Health Station, a policlinic or a hospital because of a particular health problem. The clinical diagnosis, or a diagnosis based on additional laboratory tests, will be recorded in various registers and then enters into reports to be made to higher health authorities.

In Vietnam, there exist several systems of registers and reports about infectious diseases. Firstly, there is the general health information system already mentioned in Sect. 1.2, which is managed by the Department of Planning of the Ministry of Health. It concerns non-infectious diseases as well and will be described further in Lesson 11. The routine reports in this system serve mainly to establish health statistics with a view of applications to planning and budgeting.

In addition, the National Institute of Hygiene and Epidemiology operates an information system based on the same sources of information in which the reports pass through the network of the "District Health Centres" on the district level and the "Centres for Preventive Medicine" on the province level. It concerns exclusively infectious diseases.

For certain acute infectious diseases this system foresees *monthly* reports on incidence and mortality. These are the following ones: Typhoid fever, shigellosis, amoebiasis, dysenteric syndrome, diarrhoea, viral hepatitis, meningitis syndrome, chicken pox, mumps, influenza syndrome, adenoviral disease (APC), anthrax, leptospirosis, dengue fever, rubella, tetanus, and the number of rabies vaccines used. If an outbreak occurs, these diseases should be reported immediately, and every day until the outbreak ceases.

Next, there are diseases for which *individual* notification of each case is required. The notification may be *nominative*, that is, indicating the name of the patient. The following diseases belong to this category: acute flaccid paralysis, neonatal tetanus, measles, AlH_5N_1, Japanese encephalitis, cholera and plague. In general, in addition to the diagnosis, there will be information on the patient such as age and sex, place, date of onset, profession, immunization status and exposure. Further information to be given depends on the disease. It may concern known risk factors such as lack of latrines, or observations on vectors, or a suspected source of infection, or previous or simultaneous cases around the patient. Also, the required *speed* and the means of the notification, for example by telephone or e-mail, depend on the disease in question.

For the chronic diseases tuberculosis, malaria, leprosy and AIDS, there exist in Vietnam separate special surveillance systems.

In countries that do not have an efficient information system but also for special surveillance tasks, one builds a network of so-called *sentinel stations* or *sentinel sites*. They are fixed stations that observe given health events. The underlying idea is that of sampling (see Lesson 12); instead of collecting the relevant information everywhere, one only obtains it from the sentinel stations and considers this as more or less "representative" of the situation in the whole target area. Sentinel sites may have many forms. There exists a worldwide net of "Demographic Surveillance Systems" (DSSs). In Vietnam, the "field site" in the district of Ba Vi in the province of Ha Tay belongs to it.

The main flaw of a sentinel site is that by being better equipped and managed than normal health facilities it may alter the public health situation around it, which is then no longer "typical". We will not pursue this further.

Modern epidemic surveillance is becoming a very broad subject. It is no longer restricted to the surveillance of *cases* but contains other components. They depend much on the structure of the health system of a given country. We shall not enter into details and only quote some of these additional components: surveillance of *pathogens* in order to detect mutations that might for example influence their resistance against certain treatments; surveillance of *vectors*; surveillance of the *immune status* of a population, mainly for vaccine preventable infectious diseases (serosurveillance); surveillance of *side effects* of treatments.

4.6 Outbreak Investigation and Control of Infectious Diseases

As said before, measures for controlling an infectious disease depend on its epidemiologic characteristics. We shall therefore restrict ourselves again to a few basic concepts and treat examples in Lessons 6–10.

We have already used the expressions "endemic" and "epidemic" without a definition because everybody has at least a vague idea about their meaning. Let us now make this more precise. In a given target population, an infectious disease can appear in several forms.

There may be a few *sporadic* cases once in a while. In Vietnam, whooping cough and mumps usually occur in this way.

The disease may be *endemic*, that is, cases appear regularly and permanently and the incidence remains more or less stable. In Vietnam tuberculosis, dengue fever and Japanese encephalitis are prominent examples; the plague is endemic but with a very low incidence.

An *epidemic* is a slow or sudden increase of the incidence beyond what had been considered "normal" before. Thus, in a concrete situation in order to declare that there is an epidemic, one has to fix a *threshold* value for the incidence based on surveillance of the incidence in the past. One considers that there is an epidemic as soon as the observed incidence surpasses this threshold. For example, dengue fever is nowadays endemic in Vietnam but there have also been epidemics in a recent past.

An epidemic can be restricted to a very small area, for example food poisoning by salmonella in a restaurant. It may concern a larger area up to a whole country. An epidemic that happens in a large part of the world is called a *pandemic*. The most devastating pandemic in historic times was the so-called "Spanish flu" in the years 1918–1920 with a number of cases of the order of 500 million and estimates of the number of deaths ranging from 20 to 100 million.

Let us start with a beginning epidemic, which means *outbreak investigation* and *control*. As soon as a beginning epidemic has been detected by the surveillance system, health authorities will normally form a special *task force* that could include persons outside the medical services; it is also called an *epidemic response team*. The task force may monitor the evolution of the epidemic with the help of the so-called *epidemic curve*. This is a graphic where one plots the incidence of the disease for successive time intervals, for example daily, weekly or monthly.

The team should first try to identify the source of the infection. Next, it needs to interrupt possible paths of the infection and protect persons that have not yet fallen ill. These two tasks are quite different for contagious diseases that are transmitted directly such as measles, diseases that have non-living media as their reservoir such as cholera, and diseases carried by one or several living vectors such as the plague. Let us look briefly at these three categories of diseases, keeping in mind the examples mentioned.

For directly transmitted diseases like measles, the first detected case is called the "index case". It can be the "primary" case from which the infection spreads to secondary, tertiary etc. cases. Interrupting the path of the infection may mean, depending on the kind of disease, isolation of patients and quarantine, increased hygiene, immunization of persons around the primary case, but also elimination of pathogens by disinfection. Often, this involves "encircling" the source of infection.

For cholera whose reservoir is mainly water, the source of infection is often identified by reviewing first all *possible* sources such as various parts of a river, lakes, ponds, and water pipes in the neighbourhood of the outbreak. Then, by examining them one by one, all possible sources except the "true" one are excluded. This is in fact the epidemiologic principle applied by John Snow in his historic investigation in 1853; see Sects. 6.2 and 25.1. The control of a cholera outbreak in Vietnam was described in Sect. 3.2. Another "historical" example of this method is the identification of the source of an outbreak of a hepatitis B epidemic by Wilhelm Lürman in 1883, that is, a long time before the discovery of the virus HBV; see Sect. 9.2.

Interrupting the path of infection for such diseases after having discovered the source is usually fairly obvious, depending on the situation, and we shall not enter into the technical details.

Finally, for vector-born diseases such as the plague finding the source and interrupting transmission depends indeed much on the specific features of the disease; there will be examples in Lessons 7 and 8.

Sometimes, case-control studies (Lesson 20) are being used for identifying sources of infection. A prominent example is food poisoning. The underlying idea is very simple: compare the presence of possible sources among cases on the one hand and among non-cases on the other; see the study in Sect. 3.2.

In Sect. 2.3 we have sketched the indirect effect of curative treatments on the *prevention* of infectious diseases. In a similar way curative treatments of cases can often serve to *control* an ongoing epidemic. It does so by shortening the period of time during which an infected person can infect others (infectious period). We will come back to this as well as to questions of immunization in the following lesson.

Many of the preceding remarks on control apply to *endemic* infections as well. The most serious diseases were or are the subject of a special *strategy* as discussed in Sect. 2.5. The general principles are always the same: act on risk factors, in particular by general hygiene; control the path of transmission directly, for example by controlling vectors; influence the dynamics of the transmission within the target population by immunization if possible and by curative treatments that shorten the infective periods of infected individuals. The best way to get a deeper understanding of these basic principles is to study the examples treated in Lessons 6–10.

4.7   Practical Work

1. Look at the Health Yearbooks of the Ministry of Health for the years 2000–2007. For the seven diseases dealt with in Sect. 4.2, draw simple graphs, to be designed by yourself, of the time evolution of their yearly incidence during these 8 years. Comment them.
2. Inquire at the Centre for Preventive Medicine of your province about recent outbreaks of epidemics that required special action. Then, visit a district Team for Prevention and Hygiene that had been involved and obtain a clear vision of what was done.
3. Draw the epidemic curve for an epidemic that has occurred in your commune, district or province. Influenza might be a suitable example. Decide yourself how to obtain the necessary information.

Lesson 5
Infectious Diseases: Modelling, Immunity

This lesson presents some mathematical methods and demonstrates their practical usefulness.

5.1   History

It has been observed for centuries that a patient who survives an episode of certain infectious diseases such as smallpox or measles becomes immune for life against a further infection. For smallpox, the idea therefore arose to infect persons artificially by a "mild" form of the disease. This practice seems to have originated very early in China where dried smallpox scabs were blown into the nose of an individual who then contracted a mild form of the disease and was immune upon recovery. Starting in the eighteenth century, a modified procedure named "variolation" was used in Europe. Here the dried scabs were injected under the skin.

Only 1–2% of those variolated died whereas the "case fatality", that is the proportion of deaths among those who caught the disease naturally was around 30%. However, not everybody fell ill naturally, and so the question was asked early how to *evaluate* variolation from a Public Health point of view. This was first done by the Swiss mathematician Daniel Bernoulli in 1766, who calculated its effect on life expectancy. To this end, he used the so-called statistical *life tables* that came up at that time and that the reader can find in any book on demography.

Daniel Bernoulli was the first to employ mathematical methods in Public Health beyond merely counting cases and deaths and calculating expenses. In the twentieth century one started to investigate the *dynamics* of an epidemic in a population in terms of epidemiologic concepts by applying mathematical methods. Concretely, one wanted to find the *evolution* in time of, for example, the number of "susceptibles", that is of not yet infected individuals, or the number of persons suffering from the disease, or the number of people having recovered. *Mathematical modelling* starts by representing the transition from one of these groups to another one in quantitative, mathematical terms. One then derives from it the time evolutions in question with the help of mathematical techniques. Thus, a general definition would run like this:

© Springer Nature Switzerland AG 2019

K. Krickeberg et al., *Epidemiology*, Statistics for Biology and Health,
https://doi.org/10.1007/978-3-030-16368-6_5

Mathematical modelling of an infectious disease means describing the transmission of the infection between the various groups of subjects involved (its dynamics) in mathematical terms and deducing from it the time evolution of the disease.

The first one who built such a model was the British physician Sir Ronald Ross. In 1897, he had discovered the transmission cycle of the malaria pathogen and identified *Anopheles* mosquitoes as vectors. In 1916, he developed his mathematical model for the epidemiologic features of this cycle in order to evaluate intervention strategies against malaria. In more recent times mathematical modelling was used extensively both for planning and for evaluating public health strategies including those against newly emerging infectious diseases. We have already mentioned the indirect effect of a curative treatment to prevent a disease or to control an ongoing epidemic. We will present some more examples below.

Mathematical modelling has also allowed to understand *why* an epidemic takes such and such course. For example the question of why an epidemic normally dies out before everybody has fallen ill has intrigued epidemiologists until not long ago. The standard theory up to the end of the nineteenth century was that the virulence of the pathogen decreased during the epidemic. Then, in 1906, mathematical modelling showed that this theory was wrong and that the explanation was, in a sense, much simpler. Vaguely speaking, new infections, which are required in order to keep up the epidemic can only take place if there exist *sufficiently many susceptible* subjects, and this is no longer the case when the epidemic has already lasted during a certain time.

An even more surprising result of modelling concerns syphilis cycles. In Denmark, it was already observed during the second half of the nineteenth century that, on top of an endemic component, recurrent epidemics occurred periodically every 11 years or so. Similar periodicities were found again and again in other countries and attributed to periodicities of certain social risk factors that might influence the incidence of syphilis. A long controversy ensued until in 2005 it was shown by mathematical modelling that the periodic epidemiologic behaviour of syphilis is simply due to the inherent dynamics of the disease, namely the building up of immunities in the population. Naïvely speaking, if the number of cases is increasing, more individuals become immune, which causes the incidence to fall, hence fewer persons acquire immunity, which causes the incidence to rise, etc.

5.2 Mathematical Models of the Dynamics of Infectious Diseases

In a *clinical* context, several periods concerning the evolution of a case play a role:

- The *incubation period* starts with the moment of infection and ends with the first symptoms.
- The *prodromal* phase is the period from the appearance of the first symptoms until a definitive diagnosis.

- The *sickness* period lasts from diagnosis to recovery or death. In it the disease is *fully developed*.

These three periods follow each other. In addition, one distinguishes the following two successive periods that concern mainly the *epidemiology* of infectious diseases:

- The *latent* period when the patient is already infected but not yet infectious, that is, he does not infect others.
- The *infectious* period when the patient can infect others.

The infectious period may start before or after the prodromal phase and usually ends before the disease does.

Here are some typical incubation times:

Food poisoning: some hours; cholera: some hours up to 5 days; amoebiasis: days to years, generally 2–4 weeks; influenza: 1–3 days; diphtheria: 2–5 days; dengue fever: 5–8 days; whooping cough: 7–14 days; measles: 8–14 days; tetanus: 3–21 days; syphilis: 3 weeks; hepatitis B: 40–160 days; tuberculosis: 4–12 weeks; leprosy: 9 months to 20 years, generally 4–8 years.

In order to present the essential ideas of mathematical modelling without assuming the knowledge of advanced mathematic techniques, we shall now look at an artificially simplified situation that may not be very realistic but will still display the typical features in which we are interested. We shall treat an epidemic of an acute *contagious* disease such as influenza, measles, smallpox, poliomyelitis, whooping cough or diphtheria; we may think of measles in order to have something concrete in mind. We choose a *unit of time*, for example 6 h, and start at time 0. We want to follow the evolution of the epidemic step by step where each step lasts one unit of time.

At a given moment, there exist in the target population three groups of individuals. Firstly, there is the group **S** of susceptible persons who are not yet infected but *can* be infected. In order to simplify matters we assume that an infected subject becomes immediately infectious, that is, there is no latent period. Secondly, we have the group **I** of infected people. Thirdly, there remains the group **R** of "removed" persons who have already gone through an infection and are no longer infectious. We assume that they cannot be infected again because they have *acquired immunity* which will last for life or at least for a long time span compared with the duration of the epidemic that we are modelling. For simplicity we also assume that the mortality both by the disease in question and by other causes is negligible and that no individuals are newly born within the target population. Finally we exclude immigration into, or emigration from, the population. Then the total number N of individuals in the target population remains constant, i.e. unchanged in time.

By the *dynamics* of the epidemic we mean the evolution in time of the number of individuals in the three groups and the transitions between the groups. In order to describe it mathematically, we denote by $S(t)$, $I(t)$ and $R(t)$ the number of persons in the groups **S**, **I** and **R**, respectively, at the moment t. In particular, $I(t)$ is the prevalence of the infection at the moment t. Thus

$$S(t) + I(t) + R(t) = N \text{ for every } t.$$

At the beginning, a certain number $I(0)$ of individuals got infected from outside and have become infectious. Moreover, $R(0) = 0$ because at the start of the epidemic nobody has acquired immunity from it.

Next, we note that only transitions from **S** to **I** and from **I** to **R** can occur. We need to describe them in mathematical terms. Regarding the first transition, we have already mentioned in Sect. 4.3 the concept of a *force of infection*. It is the *proportion* of susceptible people who become, on the average, infected during a given period of time of length 1. Hence the number of new infections during the period from the moment t to the moment $t + 1$ will be $S(t)$ times the force of infection in this period. It is reasonable to assume that this force of infection is approximately *proportional* to the number of possible *sources* of infection that exist at the time t, which is the number $I(t)$ of infectious individuals. Thus it is of the form $\beta I(t)$ where β denotes a certain positive "parameter" that is, at first, unknown. Therefore the number of *new* infected people during the period from t to $t + 1$ will be $\beta I(t)S(t)$.

Regarding the transition from **I** to **R**, we assume, which seems reasonable, that the number of people in **I** who recover during the period from t to $t + 1$ is proportional to the number of people who exist in **I** at the moment t. Hence it has the form $\gamma I(t)$ where γ is a positive parameter which is, again, a priori unknown. That such parameters β and γ exist is of course a simplifying assumption. Implicitly we assume here that all parts of the target population are alike regarding infective contacts and regarding the mechanism of recovery from the disease, and that people meet each other more or less at random.

Now we can compute all the numbers $S(t)$, $I(t)$ and $R(t)$ for $t = 1, 2,...$ by recurrence as soon as we give ourselves the number $I(0)$ of infected individuals at the beginning and the constants β and γ. We start by

$$S(0) = N - I(0),$$

$$I(1) = I(0) + \beta I(0)S(0) - \gamma I(0),$$

$$R(1) = \gamma I(0),$$

$$S(1) = N - I(1) - R(1).$$

Next we have

$$I(2) = I(1) + \beta I(1)S(1) - \gamma I(1),$$

$$R(2) = R(1) + \gamma I(1),$$

$$S(2) = N - I(2) - R(2),$$

and at any time t:

$$I(t+1) = I(t) + \beta I(t) S(t) - \gamma I(t),$$

$$R(t+1) = R(t) + \gamma I(t),$$

$$S(t+1) = N - I(t+1) - R(t+1).$$

In this way, we have *simulated* the epidemic mathematically. The smaller the time unit chosen, the better this simulation will be. If we replace the original time unit "1" by another one called Δt, we have to replace the constants β and γ in the equations above by $\beta \Delta t$ and $\gamma \Delta t$, respectively. There exists of course software to perform these calculations but the programming is easy and a programmable pocket calculator will suffice.

The modern theory of mathematical modelling works mainly with a *continuous* time and *differential equations* instead of the *discrete time* and *difference equations* as above but its basic ideas are the same. It handles models that represent much more general situations. Above all, it provides insights of considerable practical importance.

Firstly, it allows us to compute a number that is fundamental in most models, namely the *basic reproduction number* R_0. This is defined as the total number of new infections caused by a single infectious individual during the *whole duration* of its infectious period if the entire population is susceptible. In the particular model treated here, one can prove that

$$R_0 = N\beta / \gamma.$$

Note that this quotient does not change when we replace β and γ by $\beta \Delta t$ and $\gamma \Delta t$, respectively.

The basic reproduction number is related to the *increase* of the epidemic. From the equations above we obtain indeed

$$I(t+1) - I(t) = \beta I(t)\big(S(t) - \gamma / \beta\big).$$

Thus the number of infectious individuals increases as long as the number of susceptibles $S(t)$ is still larger than γ/β; afterwards, it decreases. At the beginning, $S(0) = N$, which means that an epidemic can only start if $N > \gamma/\beta$, that is $R_0 > 1$. This is what one would expect, but the existence of such a *threshold* value R_0 was an important discovery. It appears in many other models, too.

Secondly, the model answers the question raised in Sect. 5.1 about the part of the target population that never gets infected, that is, stays susceptible. We shall denote the number of these people by S_∞ because it is the limit of the numbers $S(t)$ after a very long time t. Then S_∞/N is the *proportion* in the target population of people who never get infected, and $A = 1 - S_\infty/N$ is the proportion of those who do contract the disease at some moment during the epidemic. This proportion A is called the *attack rate* of the epidemic. It turns out that it depends only on the basic reproduction number R_0 and can be computed from R_0 by solving for A the equation

$$A = 1 - \exp(-R_0 A),$$

which is equivalent to

$$R_0 = -(1/A)\log(1-A)$$

where "log" stands for the natural logarithm.

A third application concerns problems of immunity, immunizations and their Public Health strategies. This is the subject of the following section.

In order to simulate an epidemic with the help of the equations above, starting with a given initial number $I(0)$ of sources of infection, we need to know the size N of the whole population and the parameters β and γ. It is usually easy to estimate the size N. The two parameters β and γ can only be derived from observations. Whilst direct observations are difficult, we can sometimes exploit their relations with observable quantities. For example, it may be easier to estimate the recovery rate γ first because it is based on the observation of already existing cases. We may also use the fact that the average length of the infectious period is equal to $1/\gamma$; for measles, it is roughly 8 days. If, in addition, we can estimate the basic reproduction number R_0 from observations of many actual epidemics, this finally yields $\beta = \gamma R_0/N$. The table in Sect. 5.3 below shows the attack rate A and the basic reproduction number R_0 for some diseases of importance in Vietnam.

5.3 Immunity

In clinical medicine, *immunity* of an individual against an infection means that this individual does not contract the disease when exposed to the infection. This needs of course to be made precise in every concrete context. In this book we shall not discuss aspects of immunity which concern individual persons. They are the physiological, microbiological and biochemical mechanisms within the human body which create, maintain or annihilate immunity. Instead, we are interested in *population immunity*, that is the role of immunity in epidemiology and Public Health, for example in a strategy for preventing an epidemic in a target population.

As in the preceding section, we shall illustrate the basic general ideas in a particular situation, namely that of an epidemic of a contagious disease whose evolution is described by the simplified model presented above. There, we have introduced the parameter β, which is the average number of new infections during a unit of time *per* source of infection and *per* susceptible person. This parameter depends on many things that are partly related to each other. It depends on the *structure* of the population, for example the frequency and intensity of contacts between infected and susceptible persons. It also depends on the so-called *generation time* of the disease, which is defined as the average time between the infection of a person and the moment this person infects, in turn, a second one. Finally it depends on how easily a susceptible individual gets infected when he or she meets an infected one; this is related to his or her status of natural immunity, too. Similar remarks concern the parameter γ.

We have already noted that, even *without any intervention* from outside such as a vaccination, a portion of the target population will not fall ill. We have seen how this mechanism works: more and more individuals acquire immunity in the process of the epidemic and pass from the group **I** of infected people to the group **R** of those who have become immune. Hence there will no longer be sufficiently many individuals in the group **S** of susceptibles to uphold the epidemic, and a positive number S_∞ of them will remain susceptible forever and never contract the disease. This phenomenon is called *herd immunity* because it is *inherent* to the "herd", that is, the target population. In quantitative terms, we represent it by the proportion of people "protected" in this way, namely $S_\infty/N = 1 - A$ where A is the attack rate. Therefore it is, like A, determined by the basic reproduction number R_0.

Next we define the concept of herd immunity in the more general situation where part of the target population had been vaccinated against the disease in question. In qualitative terms the underlying idea looks like this:

Herd immunity is the fact that we need not vaccinate everybody in the target population in order to eliminate the infection from it. It represents an indirect effect of the vaccination on unvaccinated subjects.

Let us examine this mechanism more closely. To have something concrete in mind, we look again at measles and at the immunization by the current measles vaccination. To start with, we assume that this vaccination renders immune all vaccinated subjects, in other words, that its *efficacy* is equal to 100%, which is of course not true in reality.

By the vaccination *coverage p* we mean the proportion of persons vaccinated. We want to calculate the so-called *threshold coverage*, which is the minimal coverage required to prevent an epidemic. In order to do this, we model the evolution of the disease as before *after vaccination with a coverage p* and compute again its basic reproduction number. Vaccination reduces the number of susceptibles at any time and it turns out that the basic reproduction number *after* vaccination is given by

$$R_0^* = R_0 \left(1 - p\right)$$

where R_0 denotes, as before, the basic reproduction number in the original population when *nobody* had been vaccinated. This is a plausible result: the number of individuals infected by a single source during its infectious period in a completely susceptible population decreases, due to the vaccination, by the factor $1 - p$ which is the proportion of non-vaccinated persons. For $p = 0$ (nobody vaccinated), we get the same basic reproduction number as before; for $p = 1$ (everybody vaccinated) we have $R_0^* = 0$. As noted above, in order to prevent an epidemic we must have $R_0^* < 1$, which is equivalent to $p > 1 - 1/R_0$. The threshold coverage is therefore equal to

$$p_c = 1 - 1 / R_0$$

This threshold coverage p_c is also the number that must be exceeded by the coverage p in order to *eradicate* the disease. For smallpox, with a basic reproduction number of about $R_0 = 6$, one obtains $p_c = 0.83 = 83\%$. For measles, there are several estimates of R_0; if $R_0 = 15$, one gets $p_c = 0.93 = 93\%$ and if $R_0 = 20$, one has $p_c = 0.96 = 96\%$.

Recall that all of this holds under the assumption that the immunization procedure in question has an efficacy of 100%, which is hardly ever true. We have vaguely mentioned the general definition of efficacy in Sect. 2.3; let us now make it more precise. First we imagine that *nobody* in the target population was vaccinated and denote by A_1 the corresponding attack rate, which is also called the *risk* of a person in the unvaccinated target population to contract the disease. Next we imagine that, in the same target population, *everybody* was vaccinated and denote the corresponding attack rate by A_0. Then the number

$$\eta = \left(A_1 - A_0 \right) / A_1 = 1 - A_0 / A_1$$

represents the reduction of the attack rate by the vaccination in proportion to the attack rate if there had been no vaccination. It is called the *efficacy* of the vaccination. For example, $A_0 = 0$ means that $\eta = 1$, that is, perfect protection by the vaccination; $A_0 = A_1$ is equivalent to $\eta = 0$, that is, no protection at all. In short:

The efficacy of a vaccination is the proportion of individuals that are *protected* by the vaccination among those that would have fallen ill if there had been no vaccination.

We shall come back to this in the Sects. 15.1 and 18.2.

One often speaks about *vaccine* efficacy instead of the efficacy of the entire vaccination or immunization procedure. It should be clear, though, that this efficacy does not only depend on the vaccine as a substance but also on other features of the procedure, in particular on the way the vaccine is administered and on the so-called *vaccination calendar*, which indicates the age or ages of a person at which he or she should be vaccinated.

We now return to the question of an eradication strategy. If the vaccine efficacy η is smaller than $1 = 100\%$, a larger coverage will be needed, namely larger than p_c/η; this is the new threshold coverage. If $p_c/\eta > 1$, that is, $p_c > \eta$, eradication by using the vaccine in question is impossible. Unfortunately, for important diseases the vaccine efficacy η may not be well known. The principles of the methods for estimating it will be presented in Sect. 18.2. In the case of smallpox, the efficacy seems to have been near to 100% when the vaccine was applied in the successful eradication of the disease, hence a coverage exceeding 83% was sufficient. For measles, however, the estimates of the efficacy of the current vaccination procedures vary a lot, especially between developing and developed countries. A realistic value for Vietnam could be $\eta = 85\%$, which would make eradication hardly possible because $p_c = 93\%$ in the more "optimistic" case $R_0 = 15$. It is the smaller threshold coverage for smallpox, together with a longer generation time that allowed for efficient vaccination around

Table 5.1 Basic reproduction numbers

Disease	R_0	A	$p_c \cdot 100$
Smallpox	6	0.997	83
Poliomyelitis	6	0.997	83
Measles	15	0.9999997	93
Diphtheria	7	0.9991	86
Whooping cough	14	0.999999	93

new cases (ring vaccination), which explains the success of the eradication campaign of smallpox whereas measles still have not been eliminated.

Regarding poliomyelitis, its basic reproduction number depends very much on the socio-economic situation of the country in question. The value $R_0 = 6$ given in the table above refers to industrialized countries, but in some developing countries one may have values of the order $R_0 = 11$. It is also difficult to obtain a high vaccination coverage because several injections of the vaccine are needed.

Although the mathematical model of the evolution of an infectious disease described in the preceding section is indeed quite simple and to some extent unrealistic, it allows us to understand the main basic principles. They underlie all concrete situations but many additional aspects have to be taken into account when predicting the effects of a vaccination strategy and deciding about its implementation. Such aspects concern side effects as well as weighing the advantages of a vaccination against those of other strategies, in particular by economic criteria. Examples will be treated in the Lessons 6, 9 and 21.

A vaccination programme can even have a perverse effect. This happened in a European country where childhood rubella vaccination at low coverage increased the mean age of infection of adults, in particular of pregnant women, which resulted in an outbreak of the congenital rubella syndrome. This *negative indirect effect* of the vaccination had been predicted by mathematical modelling!

Table 5.1 gives typical values of the basic reproduction number R_0 and the corresponding attack rates and threshold coverage for important diseases.

In order to illustrate the phenomenon of herd immunity in a hypothetical extreme situation let us note that the attack rate $A = 0.5$ would correspond to the basic reproduction number $R_0 = 1.386$ and the threshold coverage 28%. Assuming the relatively small vaccine efficacy of 80% we would need to vaccinate only $28\%/0.8 = 35\%$ of the population in order to eradicate the disease.

Some practical aspects of vaccinations will be discussed in the Sects. 6.3, 7.2 and 22.4. In various situations measures such as better hygiene or rapid efficient treatment may be preferable.

5.4   Practical Work

Simulate an epidemic of measles with a time unit (step) of 6 h, $N = 100$, $I(0) = 1$, $\beta = 0.0045$ and $\gamma = 0.03$. Decide yourself when you will stop.

Lesson 6
Diarrhoea and Cholera

This lesson is about the epidemiology, the impact and the control of diarrhoeal diseases.

6.1 Nature, History and Descriptive Epidemiology of Diarrhoeal Diseases

Diarrhoeal diseases display several specific features. Firstly, they may be due to a very large variety of pathogens. Secondly, whilst the clinical diagnosis of the symptom "diarrhoea" is easy and standardized diagnostic decision schemes exist, for the majority of cases in Vietnam there is no laboratory confirmation of such and such agent. The percentage of hospitalized cases is relatively low; most cases are treated either at home by the family or in Commune Health Stations, policlinics or outpatient wards of hospitals. Therefore, the usual health statistics based on systematic, laboratory-based reports from health facilities can give no clear picture of the incidence or mortality by the various types of diarrhoeal diseases with the exception of bacterial or amoebic dysentery and cholera.

Thirdly, mortality is particularly high among young children. Fourth, whilst vaccines against a few pathogens were developed, until now no vaccination strategy has been generally adopted. Control of most of these diseases rests on the one hand on prevention by hygiene and on the other hand on curative strategies which are non-specific, that is, are applied indiscriminately to any of them on the basis of a clinical diagnosis. For cholera, there are in addition specific outbreak investigations and control measures as sketched in Sects. 3.2, 4.5 and 4.6.

Let us look at the main pathogens. Among the *viral* agents, the *Rotavirus* is the most frequent one; in fact, it is the main cause of severe diarrhoea in infants and young children but also frequently infects adults. It was detected in 1973. Another virus of some importance is the *Norovirus* that was found in 1968. Both are transmitted faecally-orally, mainly via food and drinking water, the *Norovirus* is transmitted also by droplets through the air.

© Springer Nature Switzerland AG 2019
K. Krickeberg et al., *Epidemiology*, Statistics for Biology and Health,
https://doi.org/10.1007/978-3-030-16368-6_6

Bacterial agents, too, play an important role. In the first place several strains of *Escherichia coli* have been known for a long time. All of them follow more or less the same path of transmission, in particular via contaminated food. Next, we have *Shigella*, especially *Shigella flexneri* that were identified in 1898 by the Japanese bacteriologist Kiyoshi Shiga as the cause of bacterial dysentery, also called "shigellosis". They are transmitted between humans by contact infections via faeces, fingers, food and flies (the "four F"). Stagnant waters are an important reservoir of the agent and a source of infections. *Salmonella* as agents of food poisoning had already been mentioned in Sect. 4.4. *Campylobacter* have their source in domestic animals, for example poultry, and water, but they can also be transmitted directly between humans; some species are a frequent cause of severe diarrhoea. Finally, there is *Vibrio cholera* to which we will come back below.

The main *parasite* at the root of a diarrhoeal disease is *Entamoeba histolytica*, which belongs to the protozoa. It causes amoebic dysentery, also called "amoebiasis". It is mainly transmitted along the faecal-oral path, with contaminated water and food as intermediate reservoirs, especially raw vegetables.

6.2   The Special Role of Cholera

Recall that the main vehicle on the route of infection by *Vibrio cholera* is water that was contaminated by infected faeces. The pathogen can enter into a dormant state and become active again later. Thus, even in the absence of cases, water which had been contaminated a long time ago can still infect food, for instance. However, Cholera is hardly communicable.

Cholera and shigellosis resemble each other regarding reservoirs and paths of infection. True, there are differences that distinguish the two diseases and their epidemiologic traits. In particular, for shigellosis, a relatively small dose of ingested pathogens suffices to produce a symptomatic case. For cholera, a large dose is required. Therefore, in a cholera epidemic adults contract the disease more frequently than children because they are subject to the risk of infection not only at home but also outside. Shigella is more concentrated on the age group 2–5 years. However, the main reason for which cholera was often singled out among diarrhoeal diseases, and in particular attracted much more attention than for example shigellosis, is neither clinical nor epidemiologic; it is historical.

Cholera has been considered a particularly dreadful disease because people remembered the great epidemics of the past. Reports from both China and India make it plausible that cholera epidemics have occurred there already in antiquity. In Europe, devastating epidemics appeared from the late eighteenth century until 1892. In Latin America, there were large outbreaks still in the 1990s and in Zimbabwe an extended epidemic took place in 2008/2009. Another heavy outbreak happened in

Haïti in the year 2010. In October 2016 a particularly vast cholera epidemic began in Yemen. According to various reports it lead until February 2018 to around one million cases and 2300 deaths and apparently did not decline at that time.

At present, cholera is endemic in many developing countries. Although the reporting on cases and deaths is certainly insufficient, one can state that mortalities are in general low. Here are the countries from which more than 100 deaths by cholera were reported in 2008: Angola 243; Democratic Republic of Congo 548; Guinea-Bissau 225; Kenya 113; Mozambique 102: Nigeria 247; Sudan 118; Uganda 120; Zimbabwe 2928. The so-called *case fatality*, that is, the percentage of all cases with a fatal issue, is around 5% in Africa and less than 1% elsewhere thanks to the curative measures described below in Sect. 6.4.

In Vietnam, too, its incidence and mortality make cholera one health problem among many others; it is certainly not the most important infectious disease. In the year 2007, there were 2.24 cases per 100,000 inhabitants in the whole country. They happened essentially in the Northern Region with 4.93 cases per 100,000 inhabitants whereas there were no cases in the Central and Southern Regions and the Highlands; see also Lesson 3.

Both preventive and curative strategies for cholera resemble those against other diarrhoeal diseases; see the following sections.

Cholera had once been called, together with tuberculosis, a *social* disease because of its great impact and because of the important role of socio-economic factors such as poverty, lack of education and poor hygienic conditions. However, this is equally true for several other diseases. For example we shall see in Sects. 23.2 and 26.2 how socio-economic factors act on cardio-vascular diseases. Thus:

The term "social disease" is now obsolete, and cholera does not play a special role apart any longer.

The study of cholera occupies an important place in the *history of epidemiology* because of the work of John Snow during the epidemic in London in 1853. He showed by purely epidemiologic means that the cause of cholera was deficient quality of water for human consumption. He published his findings in 1855. He applied them in London by removing the handle of the pump that furnished the polluted water, and no more cholera epidemics occurred there. Things went differently in the city of Hamburg, which is the largest German seaport. Its municipal authorities had the choice between, on the one hand, improving water supply and on the other hand enlarging the harbour and expanding the town hall; there was not enough money for doing both. They chose the latter and as a result a cholera epidemic in 1892 took 8605 lives. The path of infection is fairly well known and interesting. Hamburg is situated at the "Elbe" river. Water for households was taken upstream. An Asian sailor polluted the Elbe much more downstream near the harbour. However, due to the tides and particularly unfavourable winds, water containing the cholera bacteria was pushed upstream and reached the sources of drinking water.

6.3   Risk Factors and Prevention

For most diarrhoeal diseases the main risk factors can be deduced immediately from the nature of the source and the path of infection. Lacking or deficient latrines and lacking or deficient wells or other water supplies are obvious risk factors. If food is liable to be contaminated, lack of appropriate preparation is a risk factor. When there is contact transmission between persons by droplets or the four F defined in Sect. 6.1, the risk factor is mainly lack of personal hygiene. These are environmental and social factors. Risks of nosocomial infections (Sect. 1.5) are often easy to analyze but difficult to eliminate.

The preventive measures to be taken as a result of the knowledge of risk factors are also fairly obvious and well known and are usually resumed as "sanitation and hygiene". Some of them have already been listed in Sect. 2.3. Here we have good sewage, safe water supply, cleanliness and appropriate preparation of food. Typical examples for the latter would be to avoid raw milk, eggs and meat and to wash raw salads and vegetables with potassium permanganate in order to kill amoeba. Whilst sewage and safe water supply depend on economic conditions, the level of the other risk factors can be lowered by efficient health education.

Risk factors of a different kind among children that have been studied are *malnutrition* and *zinc deficiency*. They tend to increase mortality by diarrhoea. *Exclusive breastfeeding* contributes significantly to reducing mortality by diarrhoea among infants.

For two diarrhoeal diseases, namely cholera and rotavirus infections, *vaccinations* have been envisaged as alternative preventive strategies. The discussions around them illustrate very well the problems that a Ministry of Health faces before deciding which strategy to adopt. Let us look at some of the arguments.

Cholera vaccines have existed for many years. Their *efficacy* as defined in Sect. 5.2 had been estimated under controlled conditions in so-called phase 3 field trials, to be treated in Lesson 18. Efficacies of the order of magnitude of 60–85% were found. However, this protection is of very short *duration*; after 2 or 3 years it has much declined. Therefore, people living in endemic areas or areas where epidemics are to be expected would have to be revaccinated regularly and frequently, which is not only expensive but also difficult to organize. Moreover, little is known about the so-called *efficiency* of such a strategy, which means its effects *after* its implementation, especially in the long run. This is not the same as the efficacy estimated under controlled conditions in a trial. There can hardly be any doubt that in Vietnam improving hygiene and sanitation is a better strategy than to invest large sums in a regular vaccination programme. In some particular epidemics a ring vaccination around cases (Sect. 5.3) can help to control the epidemic.

In Europe, after the last epidemic in 1892, cholera was eradicated exclusively by hygienic measures.

During the last decade a certain number of vaccines against *rotavirus* infections of infants and young children were developed, tested in controlled phase 3 trials and licensed in many countries. Their *efficacy* in preventing severe diarrhoea varies; for some of them it exceeds 90%. The duration of protection is not well known up to now nor is their *effectiveness* in real settings of poor sanitation. The vaccination is also very expensive. It was recommended by WHO and in many national vaccination programmes. Side effects are rare but France recently cancelled its recommendation because of one of them.

Regarding in particular the situation in Vietnam many comments made above about cholera vaccines also apply to rotavirus vaccines. In Vietnam deaths of children by diarrhoeas caused by rotavirus infections can practically always be avoided, as we will see in the following section. Moreover, epidemiologic studies have demonstrated that children who suffer natural rotavirus infections develop immunity to subsequent infections, with the protective effect increasing with each natural infection. Therefore it is again preferable to use available funds for better hygiene on the one hand, and for improving the curative strategies on the other. Producers of vaccines exert of course much pressure on health authorities to have their products adopted.

6.4   Curative Strategies, Case-Management and Surveillance

The cause of death of patients, and in particular of children under 5 years of age, who suffer from acute diarrhoea, is almost always severe dehydration, regardless of the pathogen including that of cholera. Hence the principal aim of a curative strategy is to cure this dehydration. The case-management can start with a very simple and rapid clinical diagnosis that normally results in stating only the degree of dehydration, not the type of disease. Depending on this result, rehydration will be performed. In most cases, it will consist in drinking an *oral rehydration solution*, which is very cheap. Additional intravenous rehydration is required only in cases of very severe dehydration. We have already discussed the programme CDD (Control of Diarrhoeal Diseases) and its epidemiologic basis in Sect. 2.5. If well organized, it reduces the mortality by diarrhoea to very low levels. It has certainly been one of the most efficient and beneficial strategies in the entire history of Public Health in the whole world. In Vietnam, it is now discontinued as a special programme and its methods are integrated into normal clinical practice.

Surveillance of diarrhoeal diseases is based on the reports from Commune Health Stations, policlinics and hospitals. As said above, most diagnoses are purely clinical and thus do not differentiate between the various types of pathogens. The reports give only indicators about incidences and mortalities but do not concern single cases. Only in the case of cholera a laboratory examination and an individual notification is required; see Sects. 3.2 and 4.5. In order to get an idea of the burden of specific diarrhoeal diseases such as rotavirus infections or bacterial or amoebic dysentery special surveys are required.

6.5   Practical Work

1. Visit a large hospital in your vicinity and use its registers in order to study the incidence of, and mortality by, the main diarrhoeal diseases there during the preceding 3 months and by age groups: less than 1 year; 1–4; 5 and older. Enquire about seasonal variations.

2. Compare the epidemiology and case-management of diarrhoeal diseases of children under 5 years of age at a District Hospital with that in a Commune Health Station of the same district regarding the following criteria:

   • Definition of diarrhoea that is being used.
   • Number of cases treated per month.
   • Referrals.
   • How many patients go directly to the hospital?
   • Clinical diagnostic scheme.
   • Handling of cases that demand a laboratory analysis (which ones? where? how?).
   • Treatment.
   • Follow-up in order to find fatal outcomes.

3. Try to get a first impression of "case-management" at home (ice-berg phenomenon, see Sect. 1.3): how many cases are treated at home and how? Would it have been better if they had been handled in a health facility? To obtain such a first impression, do a very primitive "sample survey" by looking into families in your surroundings, families you know etc.

Lesson 7
Tuberculosis and Malaria

Situation, dynamics of infection, risk factors, prevention, treatment and control.

7.1 Descriptive Epidemiology

Why treating tuberculosis and malaria within the same lesson? After all, they are quite different diseases, one of them being caused by a bacterium and the other one by a parasite (see Sect. 4.1). These pathogens do not attack the same organs. The clinical manifestations and diagnostic methods of the two diseases are not the same. Their dynamics of transmission are not at all alike, tuberculosis being transmitted directly from person to person whereas malaria passes through an intermediate host. As a consequence, preventive measures against tuberculosis and malaria also differ fundamentally. Therefore in Vietnam two separate networks of services were created, one devoted to tuberculosis and the other one to malaria, each headed by a central institute in Hanoi. At present control of tuberculosis is entrusted to the "National Institute of Hygiene and Epidemiology"and malaria is being handled by the "National Institute of Malaria, Parasitology and Entomology".

However:

Tuberculosis and malaria have common features on the public health side, namely the *operational* aspects of controlling them.

First of all tuberculosis and most types of malaria are *chronic* infectious diseases. Both can be cured by drugs administered at an early stage unless the pathogens have developed resistance against them. Therefore, early detection of cases is essential. It may be done by good diagnostic practice for subjects who consult a health facility (passive case finding) or by sending out health workers into households for "active case finding" or by screening. The subsequent stages of the case-management also run along similar lines for both illnesses. Drugs will be given following a strict protocol, follow-up is important and in particular compliance with the treatment needs to be supervised; see Sect. 7.3. Such common features of the control of the two

© Springer Nature Switzerland AG 2019
K. Krickeberg et al., *Epidemiology*, Statistics for Biology and Health,
https://doi.org/10.1007/978-3-030-16368-6_7

diseases allow in principle to do much of the work by joint operations. They have motivated us to present both diseases here in one common lesson.

Let us now pass to their descriptive epidemiology and remember from Sect. 1.2:

The descriptive epidemiology of a disease rests on a clear definition of a case.

We shall look first at the descriptive epidemiology of *tuberculosis*. It is easy to follow details of the changing situation in the world by accessing the WHO Tuberculosis country profiles. In order to convey an impression of the magnitude of the problem we give in Table 7.1 below, for comparison, the incidence in the year 2016 and the mortality during 2016 in some selected countries.

The annual mortality in the whole world fluctuates around 1.7–2 million; tuberculosis causes the highest number of deaths among all bacterial infections.

For malaria the picture is a bit different from that of tuberculosis. In many countries a first diagnosis is often based on clinical symptoms only; we shall look into this further in Sects. 7.3, 19.2 and 19.3. Moreover, there may be less systematic follow-up. Available data usually represent the number of new cases reported during a given year, which means essentially *incidence* although some cases, which existed already before are reported again. Therefore some statistics explicitly assert to provide numbers of *reported cases* instead of incidences. We shall refrain from quoting uncertain figures here and only give the annual malaria incidence in the world during 2016, namely 216 million new cases, and the number of deaths in that year, namely 445,000. Nearly 90% of all cases happen in Africa. In tropical Africa, around 20% of all deaths among children under the age of 5 are due to malaria.

The preceding figures for both tuberculosis and malaria are based on those furnished to WHO by Ministries of Health. As mentioned before they depend on the definition of a case and on the diagnostic methods; see Sect. 7.3 below. They are also the results of the process of reporting indicators within the underlying information system; see Sect. 11.3. Hence they may be unreliable and different sources may give quite different figures. In Vietnam the institutes named above operate their own information systems, which are partly integrated into the general health information system of the Ministry of Health; their indicators are relatively reliable. In other countries, more precise information is only obtained by occasional surveys; a case in point is India.

Table 7.1 Incidence (unit 1000), incidence per 100,000 and mortality per 100,000 for all forms of tuberculosis in 2016

Country	Incidence/1000	Incidence per 100,000	Deaths per 1000
China	895	64	2.93
Germany	6.6	8.1	0.46
India	2790	211	33
Russia	94	66	9.4
Vietnam	126	133	15

Fig. 7.1 Recent high
malaria incidence
(incidence density) a first
visual representation by
the dotted regions

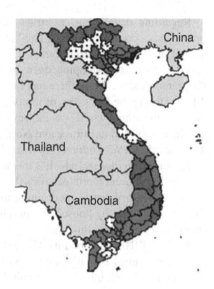

Inside of Vietnam the prevalence of tuberculosis is by and large evenly distributed over the whole country, with lower values in remote areas and higher values
in the South. Malaria has a very uneven distribution as shown in the rough map
above (Fig. 7.1) for the year 2008 where darker shades mean a higher
prevalence.

The table and the map above present the situation in various countries or regions
in a given year. They describe some aspects of the influence of the *geographical*
factor on prevalence or incidence. It is equally interesting to look at the factor
"time", in other words at *trends* in the evolution of the two diseases. Very little quantitative information exists for the time before the twentieth century, and in most
developing countries there are hardly any statistics for the first half of the twentieth
century either. The reliability of indicators from developing countries for the second
half of the twentieth century varies much between countries. Hence we shall restrict
ourselves to a few purely qualitative remarks.

Tuberculosis, especially its pulmonary form, has been one of the most threatening health problems since antiquity. It is for example described around 2700 B.C. in
Chinese and around 1500 B.C. in Ayurvedic texts. It was responsible for about one
fourth of all deaths in Europe in the seventeenth and eighteenth centuries. The mortality then declined regularly during the second part of the nineteenth century in
England and Wales, which had particularly good registers, but no doubt also in most
other industrialized countries. This was due to a change of risk factors; see Sect. 7.2.
The trend continued in developed countries into the twentieth century, especially
between the two World Wars, and became stronger with the advent of chemotherapy
around 1940; see Sect. 7.3. In the late 1980s it was reversed because of AIDS
(Lesson 10), but then there was a decrease again except in Russia and some East
European countries. At present the factor "multidrug resistance"plays an increasing
but not yet foreseeable role; see Sects. 3.3, 7.3 and 29.4.

Regarding developing countries, very few indicators are known for the time before the Second World War. The "International Tuberculosis Campaign", which started in 1948, had an important impact in most developed countries but a very varying effect in developing ones. In India, which has a "National Tuberculosis Programme" since 1962, there had been a slow downward trend until the advent of AIDS. During the last years of the twentieth century, the annual tuberculosis incidence in the whole world was increasing by a few percent each year.

Malaria existed in Europe and North America in the nineteenth century. There it was caused by *Plasmodium (P.) vivax*. This parasite can develop at lower temperatures than *P. falciparum*, which is the main pathogen of the disease in tropical countries. In Europe and North America the disease was eradicated in the first half of the twentieth century, partly by draining the breeding grounds of the Anopheles mosquitoes and partly by household spraying with the insecticide DTT. There are still many imported cases, though.

In 1955 WHO launched its "Global Malaria Eradication Programme". It rested on vector control by DDT and mass treatment with chloroquine. It was mainly implemented in South America and Asia but only little in sub-Saharan African countries. It failed, and in 1972 eradication as a goal was officially abandoned. Incidence and mortality rose again in the countries where the programme had been introduced. In sub-Saharan Africa where the programme had never been implemented, there are many highly endemic regions in which the incidence and mortality have been almost constant for many decades, and others where the disease is endemic to a lesser degree and intermittent epidemics occur. Only during the past few years, some countries could record essential success in malaria control due to the preventive and curative measures to be described in Sects. 7.2 and 7.3. In particular the incidence in whichever sense and the mortality decreased much during the last decade until 2016.

Finally, we compare the "weight", "impact" or "burden" of tuberculosis and malaria in Vietnam with each other. For simplicity, we choose again mortality as the indicator to be used for representing this "weight" although more refined descriptions exist; see Sect. 1.2. In the year 2016, mortality by tuberculosis per 100,000 people was 15 but by malaria only 0.01. Obviously, tuberculosis is a much more serious health problem in Vietnam than malaria.

7.2 Dynamics of Infection, Risk Factors and Prevention

The reader might want to start by profiting from another look at the Sects. 4.1, 4.3, 4.4 and the first two paragraphs of Sect. 5.2 for some general ideas and concepts.

The dynamics of the evolution of *tuberculosis* in a given population is not easy to investigate and to understand. There are several reasons for that. Firstly, many people are subject to a *latent infection* that may last life-long and never lead to a case of the disease. It is estimated that about 5–10% of all infected persons actually develop the disease, after an incubation time of about 4–12 weeks. Moreover, even the definition of an infected individual, that is, a case, or of a person who died from tuberculosis, is not obvious; there is no general agreement about it. Secondly, the distinction between *primary* and *secondary* tuberculosis plays an important role and so does the phenomenon of *reactivation* of a case already considered cured. Thirdly, there exist many extra-pulmonary forms of the disease but only subjects suffering from open pulmonary tuberculosis can be human sources of infection; the lung is also the usual portal of entry.

Nowadays the main pathogen of tuberculosis is *Mycobacterium tuberculosis*. Infections by drinking raw milk from cows infected with *Mycobacterium bovis* have become very rare. Thus the normal path of transmission is by droplets from man to man.

A mathematical model for the dynamics of tuberculosis along the lines of the model presented in Sect. 5.2 would be either fairly complicated or unrealistic. Hence we shall restrict ourselves to quoting only two indicators that are especially well adapted to describing essential aspects of the evolution of the particular disease "tuberculosis". The first one is the "annual risk of transmission from a single source", namely from a patient suffering from infectious pulmonary tuberculosis to other persons. It is defined as the number of persons infected per year by one source, averaged over all sources. The second indicator is the "annual infection rate". It is the proportion of the underlying population that gets infected in the course of a year. It has been estimated in many populations, either by exploiting registers or by sample surveys.

Controlling tuberculosis in a population amounts to reducing the annual infection rate, and this rate is also a good indicator for evaluating the effects of control measures. One can imagine three kinds of control measures: reducing risk factors, immunization, and treatment in order to lower the risk of transmission.

Regarding risk factors, they have been investigated extensively, starting already in the nineteenth century.

The main risk factors for tuberculosis are predisposition, that is, hereditary factors; malnutrition; alcohol; all socio-economic factors that contribute to an intensive exposition to the infection such as crowded housing; silicosis; and finally AIDS.

Recently, one has also studied social risk factors that are not *person-based* but *community-based* such as social structures and segregation between groups of people; see Lessons 24 and 26 for definitions and discussions.

Acting on these risk factors is an essential component of tuberculosis control and prevention. Regarding hereditary factors, many studies have made it likely that the predisposition to a tuberculosis infection is to some extent hereditary although the issue is less clear-cut than for the closely related disease *leprosy*; see Sect. 26.3. The obvious application is to recommend to people with many cases of tuberculosis in their family to be particularly cautious when having contacts with sources of infection and to submit to regular screening.

The most important contribution to tuberculosis control can come from influencing socio-economic risk factors. It means reducing poverty, malnutrition, poor housing conditions and the like but is of course largely outside the possibilities of health authorities. A smaller contribution could consist in education for responsible behaviour in order to reduce transmission. These are in fact the measures that have brought down the prevalence of tuberculosis in developed countries in the nineteenth and twentieth centuries.

For the risk factor HIV/AIDS, see Sect. 10.1.

Let us pass to the second kind of control measure that could be imagined, namely immunization. For a long time one has tried to prevent cases of tuberculosis by immunizing subjects, especially newborn children, by BCG (French: bacille Calmette–Guérin, introduced in 1921). This was in particular part of the Expanded Programme on Immunization (EPI) of WHO, which was launched in 1980. The effect of BCG has been the subject of much debate from the beginning. In infants it confers partial protection against a fatal issue of cases of pulmonary tuberculosis. However, this protection decreases with age and becomes small for older children and negligible for adults. Above all BCG does not prevent reactivation of latent pulmonary infection. Satisfactory protection is provided against miliary tuberculosis and tuberculous meningitis. Hence recommendations of BCG-vaccination by national health organizations usually depend on the annual infection rate in the country. For example the German Robert Koch-Institut does no longer recommend the vaccination but it is being continued in Vietnam.

Thirdly, secondary prevention (screening) and treatment as a control measure will be discussed in the following section.

The transmission process for *malaria* is characterized by the role of an intermediate host, or vector. It has the form of a cycle. A vector, namely a mosquito of the genus *Anopheles*, bites a person who is infected by pathogens of the genus *Plasmodium* and sucks his or her blood. In this way it gets infected itself. Finally it infects other human subjects by biting them and thus injecting *Plasmodia* into their blood. This is a simplified picture; the process is in fact quite complicated because the *Plasmodia* undergo various evolutions in both the vector and human. We will not enter into any more details nor list the various species of *Anopheles* and *Plasmodia* that are involved; they depend much on the geographical location.

A mathematical model of the time evolution of the prevalence of malaria is of course more complicated than the model presented in Sect. 5.2 because there are now two *reservoirs*, namely the humans and the *Anopheles*. In each reservoir there are two *compartments*, namely infected and non-infected individuals. In any case, a model consists of a system of differential equations.

Many models have been built in order to take into account aspects such as birth and death rates of the hosts, growth rates of the parasites, recovery rates and innate and acquired immunity. The Ross model mentioned in Sect. 5.1 was the first. It was of course still based on many simplifying assumptions. The essential result was to calculate an analogue R to the basic reproduction rate defined in Sect. 5.2 and to derive a corresponding *threshold phenomenon*: the disease will die out if $R < 1$. We will not give the formula for R here. It implies that in order to eradicate malaria we would have to act on the following risk factors that enter the model as parameters:

- The density of mosquitoes relative to the one of the humans.
- The average number of bites by one mosquito per unit of time.
- The probability that a bite of an infected person by a mosquito will lead to an infection of the mosquito, and analogously with the roles of the person and the mosquito interchanged.
- The recovery rate of man after an infection.
- The average life span of the mosquitoes.

This leads us naturally to the preventive measures that have in part already been mentioned. They are: reduce the mosquito populations by draining breeding grounds and spraying with insecticides; separate man and mosquitoes by appropriate clothing and bed nets; combine both methods by using bed nets that are treated with insecticides; organize an efficient system of treatment to prevent further infections (see the following Sect. 7.3). One would of course try all of these measures anyway without studying a mathematical model first, but the model provides a useful *quantitative* relation between these risk factors and the evolution of the disease.

If we want to plan preventive measures that take into account more complicated aspects of real situations, a more realistic model becomes indispensable; we can no longer just act by "good sense". This is in particular true if we need to include innate and acquired immunity in the model or to predict the effect of such and such vaccine still to be developed. The differential equations that constitute the model can then only be solved numerically with the help of a computer. It has been said that if malaria eradication will be achieved it will be first of all due to the computer!

Susceptibility to malaria is a genetic risk factor. We shall mention here a particular phenomenon, which consists in a relation between it and the hereditary disease *sickle cell anaemia* (drepanocytosis). This is a "classical" subject that has played a role in the development of the field of population genetics. One of its founders, J.B.S. Haldane, suggested in 1949 that persons suffering from sickle cell anaemia might be less susceptible to malaria. This was then first observed in 1954 by epidemiological studies in Africa. We shall come back to it in Sects. 26.1 and 26.4.

7.3   Case-Management

We are interested in those aspects of case-management that have some bearing on the epidemiology of the two diseases. Again, in order to reflect about diagnoses the first question to be answered is how to define a case. This is easy for malaria, at least in theory; it is the presence of *Plasmodia* in the blood. For tuberculosis, it is less clear-cut. A subject who had a former contact with the pathogen as shown by the Mendel-Mantoux test is not necessarily considered a case; note that about one third of mankind belongs to this category. In many medical services of the world a case of pulmonary tuberculosis is defined by the presence of *Mycobacteria* in the sputum or a positive chest X-ray examination or both. In Vietnam it is the bacteriological confirmation by the AFB-test (acid-fast bacillus smear and culture) that counts.

Hence a diagnosis may consist of a chest X-ray examination or a sputum test done either immediately or after having grown a culture of the bacilli.

To diagnose and treat a case it must be found first. Active case finding for tuberculosis in the form of screening by mass X-ray examinations had once been widely practised in several developed countries but is now rare.

For malaria, a preliminary purely clinical diagnosis still plays a role in many developing countries, for example for children by looking for an enlarged spleen. The reason is that finding *Plasmodia* by a microscopic examination of a blood sample usually takes time but a rapid treatment is considered essential. Many primary health facilities may not have a microscope and more modern rapid tests for the presence of the parasites may not be available. We will come back to this in Sect. 19.2.

We have already observed that active case finding for malaria is still being done in some developing countries; usually health workers visit households to detect cases.

Let us now look at treatments that are organized within Public Health in the form of systematic and standardized programmes. One of their main functions is to reduce the number of sources of infection and to influence in this way the dynamics of transmission.

Before 1940 practically all treatments of tuberculosis in use were inefficient in the modern rigorous sense that we shall present in Sect. 18.1. This holds in particular for all those described in the famous novel "Der Zauberberg" (The Magic Mountain) by the German writer Thomas Mann that takes place in a tuberculosis sanatorium. In 1940 the drug para-amino salicylic (PAS) was discovered in the USA and chemotherapy of tuberculosis started in 1944. It was effective where it could be applied and supervised, but often too long and costly to be used in countries with a deficient health system; the "standard" treatment lasted 18 months or more. In the early 1970s so-called *short-course* chemotherapy was first introduced. Since 1995 it has the form of the "Directly observed therapy, short course" (DOTS) defined by WHO, which lasts around 6 months and foresees to monitor strict compliance of the treatment protocol by the patient. In Vietnam it is being applied in the framework of the "National Tuberculosis Control Programme".

One of the original goals of DOTS had been to prevent the emergence of multidrug-resistant strains of bacilli. However, these have been developed recently very much in many regions, especially in India, Eastern Europe and the former Soviet Union, but also in countries possessing a good Public Health system. They present a grave menace to the whole world.

Against malaria, during many decades the standard treatment had been to give *chloroquine*. Then strains of *Plasmodia* appeared that were resistant against it. This together with DDT-resistant *Anopheles* was the main reason for the failure of the eradication programme mentioned above. A new standard treatment called "Artemisinin-based therapy" was defined. A so-called "Global Action Plan" combines the preventive measures sketched in Sect. 7.2 with case-management, vector surveillance and surveillance of resistance to drugs and insecticides; see Sect. 4.5. In some countries such as the Senegal it was fairly successful.

However, strategies need to be revised frequently. For example, a few years ago artemisinin-*resistant* strains of *Plasmodium falciparum* have appeared in the border region between Thailand and Cambodia. Also, treated bed nets were meant to deter and kill mosquitoes that are mainly biting *inside* dwellings, but in Burkina Faso a strain of *Anopheles gambiae* was discovered which was frequently infected by *Plasmodium falciparum* but active *outside*. Generally speaking drug resistance is getting steadily more frequent.

7.4 Practical Work

1. Complete Sect. 7.1 by browsing in the Internet to compare regions and trends; for tuberculosis, look also at incidence by age groups.
2. Visit the nearest tuberculosis and malaria services and try to understand the details of both their preventive and their case-management schemes.

Lesson 8
Dengue Fever

What are the characteristic traits of dengue fever?

8.1 Some General Remarks

Dengue fever shares with malaria two important traits. Firstly, its pathogen is transmitted from man to man by mosquitoes that bite and suck blood. Secondly, no vaccine exists as yet. From the point of view of case management there are two essential differences between the two diseases. Dengue is an *acute* infection; hence, follow-up plays a lesser role in its case-management than in that of malaria. Moreover, only symptomatic treatments exist. Therefore treatment is not a measure for reducing transmission by reducing the number of sources of infection; it has no epidemiologic bearing on the disease. For this reason we shall not take up the subject of its treatment.

The pathogens and the vectors were already mentioned briefly in Sects. 4.1 and 4.4. The most prominent characteristic trait of dengue fever is the existence of four different serotypes of the virus that interact with each other in various ways. This accounts for the emergence of two different forms of the disease, "mild" and "haemorrhagic" dengue fever, to be abbreviated by DF and DHF, respectively; see Sects. 8.2 and 8.3. The mild form used to be called "break bone fever" because the patient often felt as if all his or her bones were being broken. The haemorrhagic form can develop into a "shock syndrome" (DSS).

8.2 Descriptive Epidemiology

The evolution of dengue fever incidence from ancient times until now is also a characteristic trait of this disease. It was slow until a few decades ago and very rapid in the recent past. A likely case was mentioned in a Chinese medical encyclopedia in the early seventh Century. The first conclusive descriptions of a few cases in Africa, Asia and North America stem from the late eighteenth century. From that time on

© Springer Nature Switzerland AG 2019
K. Krickeberg et al., *Epidemiology*, Statistics for Biology and Health,
https://doi.org/10.1007/978-3-030-16368-6_8

until the Second World War the disease seems to have spread to many regions as ship traffic between continents became more and more intensive and carried the *Aedes* vectors with it. However, travel was then still slow and the disease appeared in the form of intermittent epidemics with intervals of 10–40 years between them. A large epidemic occurred for example in 1927/1928 in Greece.

After the Second World War, travel and transport of goods became much faster and their volume increased at a rapid pace. As a result dengue fever is now endemic or hyper-endemic in large tropical and subtropical parts of Australia, South and South-East Asia, Africa and Central and South America. Its incidence has been growing particularly fast during the last 20 years.

Reporting cases is pretty deficient in many countries. Around 2014, the annual incidence in the whole world was estimated at 50–100 million, among them 500,000 DHF cases, and the annual mortality surpassed 22,000, mainly among children. Another source mentioned an increase by around 50% of the reported annual incidence from 2010 to 2015 but attributed it to some extent to better reporting.

The factor "time" also manifests itself in the form of a seasonality of the incidence. This depends on the location but normally the incidence is high during the months of May to November with a peak in August and September.

The shock syndrome was first observed in Jamaica in 1978; at about the same time it appeared in South-East Asia. In 2006 there were roughly 500,000 cases of DHF and 20,000–25,000 deaths in the whole world; note that this implies a case fatality (number of deaths per case) of DHF of about 4–5%.

In Vietnam the first outbreak of DF was reported in the North in 1958 and in the South in 1960. By now the disease has spread out over the whole country. There were two large epidemics in 1987 and 1998. On the whole the incidence after 1998 follows an increasing trend but may fluctuate between years. For example the reported incidence was 24,430 in the year 2000, 105,370 in 2009 and 69,680 in 2011. The case fatality is less than 0.001.

The factor "age" plays an important role. People in all age groups can contract the disease. In areas with high circulation of dengue viruses such as the South, cases are mainly children under 15 years old; meanwhile in the North, with low circulation of viruses, cases include both children and adults.

The reporting mechanism on which the figures on dengue in Vietnam are based was already sketched in Sect. 4.5. Any outbreak needs to be reported to the respective "District Health Centre", which passes the information on to the Pasteur Institutes and the National Institute of Hygiene and Epidemiology and finally to the Ministry of Health. This is to be done daily. Outside of outbreaks, a weekly report is to be filed. Normally, these reports use a case definition based only on clinical symptoms but a certain proportion of suspected cases is being tested for confirmation. There are also reports within the *general* health information system to be described in Sect. 11.3.

In Sect. 4.2 we have compared dengue fever with other acute infectious diseases regarding incidence and mortality around the year 2007. In this category of diseases dengue fever was by far the most important health problem in Vietnam.

8.3 Transmission

The dengue virus is transmitted from person to person by intermediate hosts, namely mosquitoes. They belong to the species *Aedes*; in Vietnam around 96% of them fall into the group *Aedes aegypti* and the others into the group *Aedes albopictus*. They feed on human blood and this permits the transmission of the virus in both directions. Humans are almost the only reservoir of the virus in addition to the mosquitoes; monkeys and rats play a very minor role.

The *Aedes* mosquitoes are highly susceptible to the dengue virus. The geographical distribution of vectors and pathogens in the world is by and large uniform. This contrasts with the situation of yellow fever, another important viral disease that is mainly transmitted between humans by the same *Aedes aegypti* mosquitoes. However, yellow fever has never spread to Asia or Australasia. Several theories have been advanced in order to explain this phenomenon but none was generally accepted. The phenomenon remains one of the mysteries of the epidemiology of infectious diseases.

The "viraemic" (infectious) phase of an infected human during which he or she can infect a biting mosquito lasts in general around 4–5 days. This would be an important parameter if we should attempt to model the transmission process mathematically. The incubation time (Sect. 5.2) is normally 5–7 days.

Let us now have a closer look at the virus. We have already remarked that there are four serotypes, often denoted by DENV-1, DENV-2, DENV-3 and DENV-4; two more occur rarely and are mainly restricted to Thailand. In Vietnam, DENV-2, DENV-3 and DENV-1 are the most frequent ones, in this order.

The existence of these multiple serotypes has important epidemiologic implications. It leads to complicated immunologic cross-reactions in human subjects called antibody-dependent enhancement. Putting it in a pretty simplified way, a first infection by a virus of one type provides life-long immunity against a second infection by the same type, but after a certain time it may *enhance* an infection by another type. This can in particular lead to a case of haemorrhagic dengue and a shock syndrome. The probability of successive infections by different serotypes is of course higher in hyper-endemic areas with a high density of cases, and this is why haemorrhagic dengue fever has appeared only in a recent past. Also, visitors who stay only a short time in an endemic area rarely have a chance of being infected by at least two different serotypes and thus attract DHF; this form of dengue fever appears essentially among inhabitants of these areas.

This situation has made it until now impossible to develop an overall useful vaccine, in contrast to yellow fever where a vaccine of long-lasting high efficacy was developed in 1937. In 2015 a vaccine produced by the enterprise Sanofi Pasteur and called Dengvaxia was licensed in Morocco; other countries followed. It suffered from the start from a drawback common to many recently developed vaccines, namely missing information on their long-term efficacy; see also Sect. 6.3. This negative aspect is sometimes due to a short duration of trials, especially Phase III trials (see Sect. 18.4) but also to the lack of such information in generally available documents. If the period of satisfactory efficacy is relatively short, frequent revaccinations are needed and less expensive measures may be more efficient; see also the discussion in Sect. 6.3. For instance in Indonesia vaccinating one person by Dengvaxia costs over 200 US$.

However, in the particular case of dengue fever the main problem stems from the antibody-dependent enhancement described above. The World Health Organization suggested therefore vaccinating only individuals aged 9–45 years who lived in highly endemic areas and could be supposed to have already been infected. In the Philippines around 800,000 schoolchildren were vaccinated in 2016 and 2017 but an estimated 10% of them had not been previously infected. Until December 2017 there were 40 serious cases and nine deaths among the vaccinated children. The Philippine Health Department stopped the programme, returned the unused vaccines and demanded a refund for the entirety of its expenses and damages caused by the vaccinations.

8.4 Risk Factors, Prevention

When looking for risk factors, we ought to look first at the habits of the vectors. They have always been breeding in stagnant water, for example in puddles, hollow trees and other plants offering suitable cavities, but in the course of the last centuries they have adapted themselves to civilization and now use man-made water containers such as basins to store rain water, jars, flower pots, tin cans and old tyres. As a consequence, dengue fever has become above all a disease of the city although it is not absent from the countryside. Urbanization has also contributed much to the increase of its incidence during the last decades in addition to the role of travel and traffic.

We can therefore point out an obvious specific risk factor for dengue fever, namely the existence of many water containers that are not controlled for larvae of the vector. This, in turn, is influenced by more general risk factors such as overcrowding in cities, poverty, insufficient water storage systems and failing public health services. In the immediate future, however, the most effective measure of prevention is indeed a direct control of water containers. The first step consists normally of a survey of the presence and density of larvae expressed by various indices, for example the proportion of water containers in which larvae were found or the proportion of houses in which there are containers with larvae (Breteau index). Then depending on the particular situation, various stratagems may be used: eliminate superfluous containers; cover containers as much as possible; use chemicals, fish or the crustacean Mesocyclops to destroy the larvae. All of them suffer from various drawbacks. Above all they require much constant and conscientious work.

In Latin America there has been a recent attempt at predicting an outbreak and guiding preventive measures by surveying water containers by satellite.

Another method of prevention is, of course, to fight the mosquitoes directly. Thus in Greece after the epidemic mentioned in Sect. 8.2 health administrations eradicated *Aedes aegypti* completely. This seems hardly possible in most endemic countries now. Mosquito traps are being used but they also demand much work; their main role is in measuring the density of mosquitoes. If this density is high, the use of chemicals and spraying may be justified but one can never exclude with certainty negative effects on the health of people comparable to those on the health of the mosquitoes! Recently in Vietnam one has attempted to eliminate *Aedes* by infecting them with *Wolbachia* bacteria

Finally, one may try to prevent bites of persons by mosquitoes directly, for example by the use of insect repellents and suitable clothing. Mosquito nets are less efficient than against the malaria vectors because *Aedes* mosquitoes bite mainly during the day and the early morning and evening. To sum up:

At the present time controlling the larval breeding grounds is the most important measure of prevention.

In addition to the risk factors just mentioned, which are of a social and environmental nature, there are also genetic ones. For example it seems that in black Africans dengue infections are as a rule less severe than in other ethnic groups.

8.5   Practical Work

Look for *Aedes* larvae in your surroundings, and estimate the two indices defined above by organizing a small sample survey.

Lesson 9
Viral Hepatitis

This lesson describes the complex structure of the epidemiology of hepatitis B. An acute infection may lead to an asymptomatic chronic stage and this, in turn, can cause other liver diseases including cancer.

9.1 The Various Types of Viral Hepatitis

"Hepatitis" means "inflammation of the liver". Those inflammations caused by a virus present a serious problem to public health. As we have seen in Sect. 4.2, *acute* viral hepatitis in Vietnam had in 2007 an incidence of approximately 11 cases per 100,000 inhabitants. This may not appear very high. In fact, among acute infectious diseases viral hepatitis had an incidence below that of dengue fever, varicella, shigellosis and amoebiasis. Its mortality was also fairly low, namely 0.0035 per 100,000 people, that is, only one tenth of the mortality by viral encephalitis (0.0352 per 100,000). Its case fatality (number of deaths per number of cases) was $0.0035/11 = 0.00032 = 0.032\%$ compared with the case fatality of viral encephalitis, which equalled $0.0352/1 = 0.0352 = 3.52\%$. However, what makes viral hepatitis an important health problem is a trait that it shares with the human papillomavirus infection (see Sect. 22.4): it may lead to cancer. In fact an infection by the virus of the type B or C of hepatitis can turn into a *chronic* asymptomatic infection, which may entail liver cirrhosis, liver fibrosis, and hepatocellular carcinoma, often only after many years.

A long time ago hepatitis of any type was widely identified with "jaundice" (from the French "*jaune*", yellow). Jaundice was also called "icterus" from the name of a largely yellow bird. However, jaundice is a symptom that can have many other causes besides hepatitis. Later on what we now know as hepatitis A was named "infectious hepatitis" or "epidemic hepatitis" and hepatitis B was called "serum hepatitis". Early in the twentieth century one suspected already that serum hepatitis was caused by a virus. The virus HAV that causes hepatitis A was discovered under the electronic microscope in 1973 and that of hepatitis B in 1970. At the present time one distinguishes the virus types HAV, HBV, HCV, HDV and HEV. The virus

© Springer Nature Switzerland AG 2019
K. Krickeberg et al., *Epidemiology*, Statistics for Biology and Health,
https://doi.org/10.1007/978-3-030-16368-6_9

HDV is also called "deltavirus" and has only been observed as a super-infection in persons who suffer from an active HBV infection.

In Vietnam every case of any viral hepatitis needs to be reported to the District Health Centre. If there is an outbreak, a daily report must be filed; otherwise the report will be made weekly. In principle, there should always be a case investigation including a laboratory test, but in practice the reports from most health institutions are based on clinical symptoms only.

Let us first have a rapid look at hepatitis A and E, which resemble each other in many respects. Both are transmitted from man to man by the faecal-oral route, passing for example through food, water, dirty hands and flies. HEV is also hosted by some other primates. The main risk factors for both diseases are low personal hygiene and deficient water supply.

Hepatitis A appears all over the world, mainly in small outbreaks with a 2–4 weeks interval between them, especially in summer and autumn. Hepatitis E is endemic in many parts of Northern Africa, South and Southeast Asia, Eastern Europe and Central America. Floods can give rise to an epidemic. Its virus was discovered in the early 1980s in India.

Hepatitis A and E have similar incubation times of around 3–6 weeks and take a similar course although E is, on the average, a bit severer. Hepatitis A occurs mainly in children. Both illnesses are *self-limiting*, that is, the patient recovers by himself, usually in about 2 weeks except in a very few fatal cases; there is no chronic infection. Normally, no hospitalization is required. The two diseases are not a serious health problem in Vietnam.

As said above hepatitis B and C are basically different from A and E in that they frequently lead to a chronic form, to permanent liver damage, and to liver cancer. Moreover, their transmission from man to man is blood borne. There are a few differences between them, though. The virus HBV is often transmitted by sexual contacts, too, but HCV is not. Hepatitis C progresses much more frequently to a chronic infection than B; in adults, 75% of all infections by HCV become chronic but only about 5–10% of those by HBV. Moreover, there is an efficient vaccine against hepatitis B but not against C. Nevertheless the estimated prevalence of chronic HBV in the world is about twice that of HCV; hepatitis B presents the heaviest health burden among all forms of viral hepatitis. Therefore we shall now restrict ourselves to the epidemiology of hepatitis B.

9.2   History and Descriptive Epidemiology of Hepatitis B

Serum hepatitis as a specific form of hepatitis appears in medical records from the middle of the nineteenth century on. In 1883/1884 an epidemic occurred in a factory in the German port of Bremen. The physician Wilhelm Lürman whom we have mentioned in Sect. 4.6 observed that all cases took place in a particular group of people, namely in workers who were recently vaccinated against smallpox with a vaccine that had been prepared with the lymph of other people. He concluded that the disease was caused by a pathogen that could be transmitted by lymph. This was, after the work by John Snow on cholera epidemics in London published in 1855 (see Sects. 6.2 and 25.1), one of the earliest studies where the existence and mode of transmission of a pathogen could be established by purely epidemiologic means. In a sense, both investigations were rudimentary retrospective, or "historical", cohort studies as we shall define them in Lesson 17. Their purpose was to evaluate the influence of a risk factor on the occurrence of a disease. In Snow's study the risk factor was "drinking water" and his method consisted in comparing the incidence of cholera between groups of people who took their water from different sources. For Lürman, the risk factor was "lymph", and he compared the incidence of serum hepatitis between subjects who had been vaccinated with vaccines prepared by different batches of lymph or not been vaccinated at all.

Lürman published his observation in 1885 in a medical journal but apparently this was little read. Still in 1942 an epidemic occurred under exactly the same conditions, which could have been avoided. Here, some 28,000 soldiers in the army of the United States fell ill with hepatitis B after having being inoculated with yellow fever vaccine that had been prepared with human serum.

For the reasons given in the preceding section one is interested not only in the *incidence* of acute viral hepatitis B but also in the *prevalence* of its chronic form, that is in the number of people in a given population who carry the hepatitis virus of type B at a certain moment. Some people may stay chronic throughout their life; a length of the chronic period of the order of 8 years is common.

Finding the prevalence of chronic asymptomatic infections by HBV is important but difficult.

It cannot be derived from reports on new cases made by health stations and hospitals; it must be obtained from sero-epidemiologic sample surveys. Therefore, most figures given are not very precise and little can be said about the influence of the factor "time", that is, on the evolution of the prevalence in past decades.

Estimates on the basis of such surveys indicate that at the beginning of the year 2006, about 360 million people were chronically infected in the whole world. The geographical distribution of chronic HBV infection was very uneven. One distinguishes habitually areas of high prevalence defined by at least 8% chronically infected subjects, intermediate prevalence (2–7%) and low prevalence (less than 2%). By and large, the high prevalence areas comprise most of Africa except its North, China, Korea, Southeast Asia, most of the Middle East, much of Central America and some Northern parts of South America; in certain areas, there may be up to 20% chronic carriers. The prevalence is intermediate in the rest of Asia, Eastern and Southern Europe and parts of Central America and northern Latin America. It is low in Northern and Western Europe, North America, Australia, New Zealand, Mexico and southern South America.

The mortality by liver diseases due to a chronic HBV infection has a similarly uneven distribution. In the whole world, about 600,000 people die each year due to HBV-related liver diseases including liver cancer. Among people who have acquired a chronic hepatitis B roughly 40% die from its sequelae.

Vietnam is a high prevalence country.

An infection by HBV can occur at any age, but the age distribution of both the incidence of acute hepatitis B and the prevalence of its chronic form depends much on the mode of transmission, which, in turn, is not the same in all areas of the world. Hence these age distributions, too, vary between countries. We shall come back to them in the following Section.

9.3   Transmission, Risk Factors and Prevention of Hepatitis B

We have already remarked in Sect. 9.1 that the transmission of HBV can take place through blood or sexual contact. In addition, there is perinatal transmission, which is also called *vertical transmission*. In every case of transmission, body fluids containing blood are involved. Undiagnosed carriers of HBV are the main source of infection.

Contaminated blood of carriers may be transmitted to other subjects in many ways. It may happen through contaminated vaccines as in the two early examples mentioned in Sect. 9.2, or by blood and plasma transfusion, by the use of insufficiently sterilized medical instruments, by injection needles of drug addicts, by direct contact of injured blood vessels of two individuals etc.

If we want to obtain a deeper understanding of the transmission process and perhaps even model it mathematically, we need to know the probability that a given individual actually gets infected when he or she has a contact with a contaminated source. To have something concrete in mind let us think of a contact in the form of an injection by a contaminated needle. We have already discussed probabilities of this type in Sect. 4.3. In Sect. 7.2 we were looking for the probability that a person who is bitten by a Plasmodium infected Anopheles will attract malaria. Unfortunately, there is no universally accepted name for these probabilities. They are frequently called "infection probabilities" or "infection risks", more precisely infection risks *per contact* or *per exposure*, but also "transmission risks" etc. It is interesting to note that for HBV they are much higher than the corresponding probabilities for HIV (see Sect. 10.4). Depending on the form of contacts they are equal to 3–30% as compared with a transmission risk per exposure of the order of 0.3–0.7% for HIV. In particular the transmission probability in unprotected sexual contacts of various forms is mostly around ten times higher for HBV than for HIV.

In Southeast Asia the predominant route of transmission is *perinatal* with high transmission risks. Depending on the status of the infected mother, the probability that she will infect her child at birth varies between 20 and 90%. Also, as stated in the preceding section, the prevalence of chronic carriers is high, and this is true in particular among mothers. These two facts together imply that the incidence of infections is especially high among young children.

If a person suffers from an acute hepatitis B, the risk of passing to the chronic stage is, all ages taken together, of the order of 5–10% as we have observed in Sect.

9.1. It depends, however, very much on the age at which the acute infection occurs. For infections in adults and older children it is less than 5%, in younger children it hovers about 70% and for infections acquired at birth it is about 95%.

Thus the transmission mechanism is complex, but knowing it in broad outlines we can nevertheless derive the main risk factors. In low prevalence areas, drug addicts using injection needles, male homosexuals and certain categories of health care workers are at high risk. Prevention therefore consists of appropriate health education, needle exchange programmes for dugs addicts and selective vaccination of health care workers. Screening for HBV of blood donors and of products to be injected is of course also essential.

In Southeast Asia the main risk factor is having had an infected mother. Therefore, the main preventive measure is vaccinating infants as early as possible, preferably within a systematic strategy such as EPI (Expanded Programme on Immunization). The present HBV vaccine has an efficacy of over 95% during a long time.

We have already pointed out several times that systematic curative or preventive treatment of people for an infectious disease has effects not only on the individuals treated but usually also has, by reducing the number of sources of infection, an *indirect* effect on the entire population in which it takes place. It is desirable to predict such an indirect effect in a quantitative way. There is no curative treatment of hepatitis B but preventive measures such as vaccinations exist. One would for instance like to decide about the best vaccination strategy, taking into account elements such as the cost of vaccination or possible side effects. For this, mathematical models are needed. Several models for hepatitis B have been constructed and evaluated. They are necessarily complicated because of the complex nature of the transmission process.

9.4   Practical Work

Inform yourself about the details of the practice of a province hospital for diagnosing and reporting acute and chronic hepatitis B and C. Regarding the chronic form, its prevalence is sometimes being estimated *indirectly* by using the long-term sequel as a source of information; find out whether this is being done in the hospital you are visiting.

Lesson 10
HIV/AIDS

The epidemiology of HIV/AIDS is determined by several particular traits of the disease. Its mechanism of transmission resembles that of hepatitis B. During a long and almost asymptomatic period the virus destroys the immune system of the infected subject, who finally dies of opportunistic infections. There is no vaccine. Treatment is problematic but has recently made progress.

10.1   History and Typical Traits

The disease called AIDS (Acquired Immunodeficiency Syndrome) results from an infection with either of two retroviruses, HIV-1 or HIV-2 where HIV stands for "Human Immunodeficiency Virus". The first one is by far more frequent and has caused a pandemic. For simplicity, we shall restrict ourselves to looking at the epidemiology of this infection only, and always write HIV to mean HIV-1.

In contrast to all other health problems studied in this book except traffic accidents, AIDS is an *emerging* disease, which has only a short history as a human illness. It is likely that HIV has existed in chimpanzees for a long time and was introduced into human populations in Africa around the mid-twentieth century. In the year 1981, 5 cases of a rare form of pneumonia and 26 cases of a rare tumour, Kaposi's sarcoma, were identified in the USA among homosexual men, and public health officials soon found evidence that they were connected with a deficient immune system of the patients. A first definition of this deficiency syndrome was given in 1982 and later expanded. In 1983 a group of scientists at the Pasteur Institute in Paris headed by Luc Montagnier isolated the causative virus from lymph nodes of a patient. In the following year Robert Gallo and his collaborators in the USA confirmed the discovery of the virus and showed that it actually caused AIDS.

In Vietnam, the first infection by HIV was diagnosed in December 1990 in Ho Chi Minh City.

The main characteristic trait of an infection by HIV is a slow and long progression through a chronic and asymptomatic phase to various opportunistic diseases due to a loss of immunity. They finally cause the death of the patient.

© Springer Nature Switzerland AG 2019
K. Krickeberg et al., *Epidemiology*, Statistics for Biology and Health,
https://doi.org/10.1007/978-3-030-16368-6_10

In contrast to hepatitis B, the transition to the chronic phase takes place in practically *every* case of an infection by HIV, and this phase almost always leads to the various diseases that will eventually kill the patient. AIDS means the occurrence of these diseases whereas the notation HIV/AIDS stands for the entire process from the beginning of the infection to the end.

Let us look in detail at the "natural history" of a case. We shall not treat the virological details but only the facts that are essential for understanding the epidemiology of HIV/AIDS and for applying it, in particular to surveillance. During the entire progression of the disease the state of the patient can be described by, among others, two quantities, his viral load and his CD4⁺ T-cell count. The viral load is defined as the number of viruses (HIV RNA copies) per cubic centimetre of blood plasma. The CD4⁺ T-cell count is the number of CD4⁺ T-lymphocytes per cubic millimetre of blood. It represents the strength of the immune reactions of the patient; values between 500 and 1600 are considered normal.

We shall see in Sect. 10.4 how the virus can enter the body of an individual and thus start the infection. Its first phase is the acute "primary" HIV infection, which usually lasts several weeks up to 6 months. It is mostly asymptomatic except certain influenza-like symptoms in some patients. The viral load is rapidly increasing whereas the CD4⁺ T-cell count decreases from its initial normal value to something like 300. At the end of the first phase the viral load may decrease briefly and the CD4⁺ T-cell count increase again, but then, during the long second phase of chronic infection and clinical latency the original trend is restored: increasing viral load and decreasing CD4⁺ T-cell count.

During these first two phases the HIV-infection can be ascertained by an HIV-*test*. Such a test either detects the virus itself or the presence of antibodies, that is, of "seroconversion", in serum, saliva or urine of the subject. Nowadays several tests exist and are being used alone or in combination with each other. We shall discuss them further in Sect. 19.2.

Finally, the third phase of the history of a case is that of AIDS. It begins with the first constitutional symptoms that affect the general wellbeing of the patient when the CD4⁺ T-cell count drops below 400. Opportunistic infections appear when it falls below 200. The "waiting time" from the primary infection until the beginning of AIDS is on the average 8–10 years but values of about 20 years have been observed. The only known risk factor for a more rapid progression to AIDS is age; progress is faster in older subjects.

Opportunistic infections are the most visible elements of AIDS. We have already mentioned Kaposi's sarcoma, which is caused by the human herpes virus 8. Burkitt's lymphoma is another example; it results from an infection by the Epstein–Barr virus. Note that the concept of an opportunistic infection is a purely epidemiologic one. It means that the infection itself or a grave consequence such as cancer has a significantly higher incidence among HIV-infected subjects than among non-HIV-infected people.

The principal opportunistic infection is nowadays tuberculosis. Its active form appears already at higher CD4⁺ T-counts than all other opportunistic infections. As a result, HIV has become the main risk factor for developing active tuberculosis and is responsible for a strong increase of its incidence. Tuberculosis also *progresses* more rapidly among HIV-infected persons. It is the leading cause of death among them.

Hepatitis B as an opportunistic infection presents a similar picture. The probability of passing from the acute to the chronic stage is much higher among HIV-infected persons than among non-HIV-infected ones. The same is true for developing cirrhosis and for death from liver disease.

The Centers for Disease Control and Prevention (CDC) in the USA published a list of 27 opportunistic infections, so-called "AIDS-defining clinical conditions", which is widely used in surveillance and diagnosis.

10.2 Surveillance

Surveillance of HIV/AIDS in a target population consists in estimating regularly the incidence of primary HIV-infections (number of new infections during a given period, for example a calendar year), the prevalence of chronic infections (number of existing infections at a given date) and the incidence and prevalence of AIDS. In practice, surveillance is largely combined with finding and keeping track of infected subjects and of subjects suffering from AIDS, the ultimate goal being to treat them. The methods of surveillance are determined by the "natural history" of cases as described in the preceding section.

In Vietnam, most subjects suffering from AIDS will soon seek treatment in a policlinic or hospital where their disease will be correctly diagnosed and recorded. They will normally be followed during the whole duration of their illness. Hence:

The incidence and prevalence of AIDS in Vietnam can be obtained from the relevant reports in the health information system. This allows the health services to monitor their trends over time.

By contrast, frequencies of HIV-infections are not easy to obtain:

It is difficult to monitor the incidence of primary infections and the prevalence of chronic infections *before* the beginning of AIDS.

There are three reasons for it. Firstly, these infections are mainly asymptomatic, which implies that patients do not seek contact with the health system (iceberg phenomenon). Secondly, even individuals who suspect that they are infected because of, for example, unprotected male homosexual contact often hesitate to submit to a test. Thirdly, active case finding by screening with the help of appropriate tests cannot be organized in the entire population. Therefore:

The *prevalence* of HIV-infections at a given date is estimated by sample surveys.

In such a survey, the sampled subjects are submitted to one of the HIV-tests mentioned above. A sample survey provides an estimate of the prevalence in the target population from which the sample was drawn; see Lesson 12 on how to organize them.

Ideally the target population would be the entire population of, for example, a province or a country. Such surveys would be expensive, though, and were soon considered unnecessary. In fact from the evolution of the disease since the early 1980s, certain risk groups became known where most cases occurred (see Sect. 10.4, below), and hence most sample surveys or even screening programmes took place in these groups. This included surveys among all new-borns. However, more recently, in several countries there have also been many cases among people who do not belong to any known particular high risk group; thus sample surveys in these risk groups alone are not sufficient. In Vietnam sampling makes use of HIV-sentinel sites, too; see Sect. 4.5.

Finally, finding the *incidence* of HIV-infections can be treated as a purely mathematical-statistical problem. We have already remarked that the incubation period from the primary infection to the diagnosis of AIDS lasts on the average 8–10 years. From many studies one knows not only these average values but also how the values of the incubation time are spread around them, in other words, the so-called *distribution* of the incubation time; for a closer look at the concept of the distribution of data, see Sect. 13.2. Since almost every HIV-infection eventually leads to AIDS it is not surprising that the incidence of HIV-infections can be calculated from observed incidences of AIDS if we know the distribution of the incubation time. The method for doing this was especially developed for the study of the epidemiology of AIDS under the name "back-calculation". It is fairly elementary and similar methods had already been employed before for tuberculosis. Summing up:

Incidences of new HIV-infections are obtained from observed AIDS-incidences by back-calculation.

10.3 Descriptive Epidemiology

In the preceding section we have seen how indicators for the distribution of HIV/AIDS are found. The process involves registration of cases, sample surveys, screening, reports within a health information system and calculations. These operations do not function to perfection in all countries. Hence the final figures that are published by Ministries of Health and UNAIDS (The Joint United Nations Programme on HIV/AIDS) are not always reliable. UNAIDS therefore also provides lower and upper limits between which the true indicators will be situated with high probability. For example, for Vietnam, the prevalence of HIV-infections in 2016 in the whole country is given as 250,000 cases but with a lower limit of 220,000 and an upper limit of 290,000, which means that the figure 250,000 is uncertain, indeed. For the concept of a *confidence interval* that is related to this practice, see Sect. 14.3.

The distribution of the disease over the world is very heterogeneous. In the early years of the pandemic one distinguished three areas defined by "patterns", that is, the occurrence of cases in various risk groups. Patterns I and II are assumed to have developed already in the 1970s. According to Pattern I, HIV spread among homosexual and bisexual men and intravenous drug users. This happened in Western Europe, in parts of Latin America and in North America. Pattern II meant that heterosexual individuals of both sexes were infected. This took place in Sub-Saharan Africa and parts of the Caribbean. Pattern III covered, in the 1980s, Asia, Eastern Europe, the Middle East and North Africa. Here, only imported cases from Patterns I and II areas existed.

At present, the situation is quite different. Roughly speaking, both Patterns I and II have spread to the whole world although in varying proportions; there are no more Pattern III areas. Let us look at the year 2016, using figures provided by UNAIDS, and start with the global indicators. The prevalence of HIV-infections at the end of the year 2016 in the whole world was about 36.7 million, its incidence in that year was 1.8 million, and the mortality from AIDS in 2016 was one million, less than the mortality from tuberculosis.

As said above, these figures are estimates and not overly reliable. From the description of the estimation processes made in Sect. 10.2 it is fairly clear that the estimates of incidences of HIV-infections are the least reliable ones. In fact, for the global incidence in 2016 a lower limit of 1.6 million and an upper limit of 2.1 million are given; they are far apart.

Next, we outline the influence of the geographical factor by Table 10.1. It was obtained by modifying slightly a table by UNAIDS, in particular by omitting lower and upper limits.

We see that incidences and mortalities in this table are by and large of the same order. This reflects the fact that, in a more or less stable situation, most HIV-infected subjects eventually die of AIDS.

In order to assess the importance of the HIV-problem for a given region, one would of course also have to calculate the corresponding *densities*, that is, the prevalences, incidences, and mortalities of the table below divided by the number of inhabitants of the areas in question; see Sect. 15.1.

Table 10.1 Prevalence and incidence of HIV-infections, mortality from AIDS, by area and for Vietnam, in 2016. Unit: 1000 individuals

Area	Prevalence	Incidence	Mortality
Eastern and southern Africa	19,400	790	420
Western and central Africa	6100	370	310
Middle East and North Africa	230	18	11
Asia and the Pacific	5100	270	170
Latin America	1800	97	36
Caribbean	310	18	10
Eastern Europe and central Asia	1600	190	40
Western and central Europe and North America	2100	73	18
Whole World	367,000	1800	1000
Vietnam	250	11	8

There may be great discrepancies also *within* regions. For example, in Sub-Saharan Africa, most southern African countries are more exposed than those further to the north. In Oceania, Papua New Guinea has a particularly high prevalence. In Vietnam there are HIV-infected people in all provinces.

Regarding the factor "sex", there is globally no important difference between women and men. The prevalence of the infection among women in the whole world in 2016 was about 17.8 million, that is, 48% of the total prevalence. However, in Africa about two thirds of infected people are women. This is the result of the transmission of the infection by heterosexual contacts; we shall come back to this in the following section. In Vietnam among adults aged at least 15, only 27% of all infected persons are women.

"Age" is an important factor, too. Globally, the infection strikes above all young, sexually active adults but also children. We shall restrict ourselves to distinguishing between children, defined by an age under 15, and adults, aged at least 15, and present indicators as percentages of figures for children among the corresponding figures for the two age groups together. In the whole world, the prevalence of HIV-infections in 2016 for children was about 6% of that of the prevalence for all people, the incidence in 2016 was, correspondingly, 9%, and the mortality was 12%.

There are again enormous regional differences. They appear even more striking when we use the division of the world into "areas" as employed by UNAIDS in the year 2006. We shall give only three characteristic values for that year. The percentage of the prevalence in children among the prevalence in all subjects was 8% in Sub-Saharan Africa, 3.5% in South and Southeast Asia and 0.4% in Western and Central Europe. Again, this is connected with the transmission pattern, to be discussed in the following section. In Vietnam in 2006 there were about 2–3% of children among HIV-infected persons.

Finally, let us cast a glance at the factor "time", that is, at "trends". We start with the year 2007. The reader can then use the situation at that moment to assess the situation in later years. Worldwide, the prevalence was still increasing. It was estimated at 29 million in 2001 and at 33 million in 2007; recall from the Table 10.1 that it is about 37 million in 2016. Regionally, the picture varies a lot. In Sub-Saharan Africa, the prevalence decreased substantially in some countries, for example in Senegal, which implies that it has started declining slowly for the area as a whole. In Asia, the incidence in 2007 was higher by about 20% than in 2001; as a consequence the prevalence was still increasing. This trend was particularly pronounced in Indonesia. By contrast, the prevalence was diminishing in Cambodia, Myanmar and Thailand. This is most likely both the result of preventive measures (Sect. 10.4) and the indirect effect of treatment (Sect. 10.5). The same holds for Western and Central Europe and North America. In Vietnam the prevalence increased from about 222,000 in 2003 to 290,000 in 2007 and then decreased to 250,000 in 2016.

10.4   Transmission, Risk Factors and Prevention

For a more precise description and prediction of the transmission process in a population, in particular through mathematical modelling, the *infection risk* or *infection probability* plays an important role. We have already mentioned it, for example for malaria in Sect. 7.2 and for hepatitis B in Sect. 9.3. It is the probability for a subject to get infected in a contact with an already infected person. Obviously, this probability depends not only on the type of contact but also on the viral load of the already infected person. The infection risks as given for various types of contact are therefore *average* values. They have been estimated through many studies.

HIV/AIDS is a *blood-borne* disease. We have discussed "paths" or "patterns" of transmission in a general way in Sect. 4.4. For the HIV they look like this:

There exist four paths of transmission: directly through blood or blood products; by homosexual contacts between men; by heterosexual contacts; from mother to child.

Let us have a closer look at these ways of infection, keeping in mind that they may change gradually in the course of time.

Direct transmission through *blood* or *blood products* happens among injecting drug users when they share infected needles and syringes. In the 1980s, many people in many countries, especially haemophiliacs, were also infected by the transfusion of infected blood as part of a medical treatment. A person injecting a drug by a needle that had been employed before by an infected drug user will become himself or herself infected with a probability of the order of 0.003–0.007 (0.3–0.7%). The risk of getting infected through a transfusion of infected blood is much higher, namely around 90–100%. Injecting drug use accounts for an important part of infections in Eastern Europe including Russia and Ukraine and in Central Asia. In China for a long time it caused the majority of infections but now other sources contribute much, too; see the end of the following paragraph.

The other three ways of infection pass through mucosal membranes and involve semen, vaginal fluids and breast milk. *Homosexual* contacts between men still play an important role in Central and Western Europe and North America. Infection through *heterosexual* contacts is gaining more and more importance in many countries, for example in Central and Western Europe, and is by far the most frequent one in Sub-Saharan Africa. In Australia and New Zealand most new infections occur in prostitutes; in China, the prevalence of the infection in this group is also high.

The infection risk in sexual acts depends much on the type of contact. Receptive partners are in general at greater risk than insertive ones. In particular in heterosexual intercourse the risk for the female partner of an infected man is higher than that for the male partner of an infected woman; these risks are of the order of 0.01–0.15%. This fact, together with the predominant role of heterosexual transmission in Sub-Saharan Africa, explains the high proportion of infected women in that region mentioned in the preceding section. The highest risk of infection, about 3%, is attached to receptive anal sex. Anal sex is often the main method of birth control, especially in Africa, which aggravates the problem.

The fourth type of transmission is from *mother to child*. It can happen during pregnancy, labour and through breast-feeding. The infection risk for the baby of an infected mother is high, of the order of 25–40%, of which nearly half is due to breast-feeding. Hence the prevalence of the HIV-infection is connected with the prevalence among women on the one hand and breast-feeding practices on the other. This accounts in particular for the large number of infected children in Sub-Saharan Africa.

Knowing the paths of transmission it is easy to guess what the main risk factors are. Firstly, there is sexual intercourse of any kind with partners who might be infected, unless a protection, usually in the form of a condom, is being employed. Secondly, there is the reuse of needles and syringes for injecting drugs. Thirdly, there is giving birth and breast-feeding by an infected woman.

In addition to these obvious risk factors, many others, less obvious, have been studied. In particular, for sexual contacts there is a long list of diseases of the infected or the "susceptible" partner that increase the infection risk.

Social risk factors, too, have been investigated extensively. Education and profession play an important role. Sometimes the results of such studies are quite unexpected. For example it was generally assumed that in infected couples where the husband had often been away from home for a long time for professional purposes (migrant workers, truck drivers etc.), it was always *he* who gave the infection to his wife. In a recent study in South Africa, however, in about one third of all infected couples it was the woman who had been infected first.

Preventing a disease means, in the first place, acting on risk factors. If one looks at the risk factors described before, one preventive measure comes immediately to mind, namely health education.

One of the main strategies to prevent HIV/AIDS is intelligent health education.

For example, the use of condoms, both male and female, needs to be promoted. For injecting drug users, in many countries there exist needle exchange programmes; they have to be advertised well etc. At any rate, education must not be confined to only *enumerating* various measures or to trying to impose ill-defined "moral" sexual behaviour. Health education about HIV/AIDS was treated extensively in the book [2] of the series "Basic Texts in Public Health"; see the description of the series at the end of the present book, which is the 2nd edition of its volume [1].

Male circumcision was advocated as a measure for reducing sexual HIV-transmission. On the basis of many observational studies (see Sect. 15.3) UNAIDS and WHO concluded in 2007 that under certain circumstances it reduces the risk of infection of men in heterosexual contacts. However, they should still use other methods of prevention. Moreover one might fear that circumcised men, feeling themselves "protected", will resort to increased sexual activity, which offsets a possible protective effect. Besides, circumcision is not feasible everywhere. More recent studies found no effect on the risk of infecting men in homosexual contacts or when engaging in anal sex of any form.

Vaginal jellies containing an anti-retroviral substance to be applied before intercourse have been submitted to many trials, for example in South Africa. The main problem that arose was "no compliance": many women in the "treated" cohort claimed to have applied the product all the time but in fact had not done it. No study found a risk reduction over 50%.

Regarding mother to child infections, we can say:

Preventing mother to child transmission is a particularly complex problem.

The two types of interventions described below concern already *infected* mothers. Hence their first step is to recognize the serostatus of pregnant women. To this end, an HIV-test must be offered to all future mothers or at least to those from high-risk groups. Then, the infection risk during pregnancy and labour can be reduced by giving the infected mother certain antiretroviral drugs. A similar approach to control the transmission by breast-feeding requires giving a drug over prolonged periods, which poses various not yet quite elucidated problems. Radical solutions such as systematic caesarean deliveries or no breast-feeding at all are obviously not to be generally recommended either.

Next:

There is no vaccine to prevent the infection by HIV.

Let us finally recall once more that a curative treatment of an infectious disease, by reducing the number of sources of infection or their infectious periods, usually also has an indirect effect on the incidence of the disease and may be an effective measure of prevention. Until a short time ago such an indirect effect on HIV-infections was hardly taken into account when planning strategies to control the disease but recently mathematical models to predict it were published. This brings us to the last section of the present lesson.

10.5 Case Management

Let us repeat a banal remark: in order to be treated, an HIV-infection must be known. The treatment should start *before* the AIDS phase. Hence case management begins by offering an HIV-test to all members of high-risk groups or to the entire population. This must be preceded by solid and efficient health education measures that make the availability of the test known and present its advantages in a clear and vivid fashion. Some more details on *screening* for the infection will be given in Sect. 19.3.

A first antiretroviral drug, AZT (an abbreviation of its name in chemistry), also called Zidovudine, was licensed in 1987 in the USA. It had originally been developed as a possible anticancer agent. Its immediate purpose was to reduce the viral load and to increase the CD4$^+$ T-cell count of the patient. Further studies showed that it did this only imperfectly. Also, resistances and side effects appeared. At present, around 25 such drugs exist and are being used alone or in combination. In 1996 a particular combination of three drugs called HAART (Highly Active Anti-Retroviral Treatment) was introduced and is now being widely used. It reduces the viral load, but does not eliminate the infection completely. Latent infections in some cells can later give rise to new general infections, often after decades, and therefore HAART needs to be applied lifelong.

As in the treatment of other chronic infectious diseases, for example tuberculosis (Sect. 7.3), the *adherence* by the patient to the treatment rules, also called *compliance*, is often difficult to achieve. These rules are complicated, requiring daily injections and intake of pills, and restrictions on food. Moreover, side effects are frequent and sometimes severe. It is therefore difficult to predict the influence of a HAART programme on the evolution of the disease in a given country. Also, drug resistances are emerging. Finally, cost and the general state of the health system of the country play a crucial role. To resume:

Systematic treatment as a public health measure is to a large extent a matter of good organization and funds.

In Vietnam in 2016 the estimated coverage by antiretroviral therapy of HIV-infected people was 47%.

In addition to the problem of treating the HIV-infection itself, there is also the question of how to treat *both* the infection and such AIDS-defining illness. For example for tuberculosis, according to recent studies it seems to be advisable to start the treatment by anti-retroviral drugs about 2 weeks after the beginning of the treatment of tuberculosis as described in Sect. 7.3. This is an even more difficult problem for public health.

10.6   Practical Work

1. Compute, for all geographical areas of the Table 10.1, the prevalence divided by the incidence. Think about possible explanations for a high or low value, respectively, of this quotient.
2. In the same table, compare the incidences with the mortalities and try to interpret the results. What could be the reason for the deviating situation in the two European areas plus North America?
3. Study and describe in concrete details the reporting process on HIV/AIDS in a Vietnamese province: reports on new cases, on the follow-up of patients, calculation of incidence and prevalence of HIV-infections and of AIDS. Which methods are being used?
4. Among all infectious diseases in Vietnam, would you regard HIV/AIDS as the main health problem, or as one of high importance among others, or of average importance or of minor importance? Define yourself your criteria.
5. This is a question that concerns the Lessons 6–10 together: which of the diseases described there are communicable and which ones are not (see Sect. 4.1).

Lesson 11
The Origin of Information: Registers and Health Information Systems

This lesson describes permanent sources of data and of epidemiologic indicators that are derived from data, in contrast to non-permanent data collection organized for a particular purpose within a particular study. It starts with a section on the underlying basic concepts.

11.1 Units, Variables, Data and Indicators

Let us go back to Lesson 1 and in particular to Sect. 1.2 and have another look at the Register of Consultations of a Commune Health Station. In order to explain the basic ideas we reproduce below, as Table 11.1, a very simplified version of a page of this register. The columns "Insured or free of charge", "Profession", "Ethnicity", "Place of treatment", "Person consulted" and "Remarks" were omitted and others modified; in particular the entries for "symptoms" and "treatments" were drastically shortened.

Here, each *row* corresponds to a consultation. Each consultation is called a "unit" of the register. The units are numbered. Other registers in a Commune Health Station have other units. For example, there exists a register of births where each row corresponds to a delivery in the commune; in that register a unit is a delivery.

Next, let us look at the *columns* of the register above, for example the column "age". For each unit, i.e. for each consultation, we find here a particular value, namely the age, given in years, of the patient who consulted. Thus, this value depends on the unit. It is a *variable* in the sense that we have already illustrated but not yet rigorously defined in Sects. 1.4 and 1.5. We shall now state the general definition of the concept of a variable:

For a given set of units, a variable attributes a specific value to each unit.

Thus, in mathematical terms, it is a *function* defined on the set of units. We have to distinguish clearly between the *variable* "age" and the age of a *particular* patient, for example the age "71 years" of the person in the consultation (unit) no. 2.

The values of the variable "age" are numbers; in the example above they are the numbers 4, 71, 19 and 34. The values of all other variables in the register such as

© Springer Nature Switzerland AG 2019
K. Krickeberg et al., *Epidemiology*, Statistics for Biology and Health,
https://doi.org/10.1007/978-3-030-16368-6_11

Table 11.1 Register of consultations (excerpt)

Number	Name	Sex	Age	Address	Symptoms	Diagnosis	Treatment
1	Nguyen Van Anh	M	4	Hamlet 3, commune Nghi Cong, district Nghi Loc, province Nghe an	High fever, cough, thorax shrunk, Nt > 50 l/p, ...	Bronchitis, pneumonia	Cepotacime, paracetamol, mandarin orange juice, honey, ...
2	Nguyen Thi Hoa	F	71	Hamlet 4, ...	Wheezing, whistling, cough...	Asthma bronchiale	Various drugs
3	Nguyen Thi Nga	F	19	Hamlet 5, ...	Stomach-ache, appendix both sides swollen and aching	Appendicitis	Various drugs, solution for female hygiene
4	Nguyen Van Mui	M	34	Hamlet 3, ...	Cough, coughing up much phlegm...	Chronic bronchitis	Various drugs

"name", "sex", "address" and "symptoms" are not numbers but letters or words. In order to allow a statistical treatment as discussed later in Lesson 13, they must be transformed into numbers by *coding*. The variable "sex" is particularly easy to code, for example by representing the male sex by 0 and the female by 1. However, in a register at the primary level such as the register of consultations above is not practical to use coded versions for all variables when they are recorded first by the health staff. It would be too abstract and errors would be much more likely to occur. Instead, in a good system of registers, there should be rules for writing addresses, symptoms, diagnoses and treatments in a way that makes their coding easy if needed for a statistical analysis. The first exercise of Sect. 11.4 is meant to illustrate this idea.

The values of variables are commonly called "data". They are the "entries" in the boxes of the register. Thus we see that the outlay of a register such as the one above has a clear logical structure:

The rows (lines) of the register correspond to the units, the columns to the variables and the boxes to the data.

The logical structure of a register stored in a computer is exactly the same. As in a "paper-based" register it is important to distinguish clearly between these three concepts: units; variables; data. Entering data in a form that makes automatic coding possible becomes particularly important.

Now, what is an *indicator*? Some people confuse indicators with data or with "parameters". Let us start with three examples of indicators from the register above:

I_1 is the proportion of women among the patients, that is, $I_1 = 0.5$.
I_2 is the average age of the patients, that is, $I_2 = 32$.
I_3 is the average age of the female patients, that is, $I_3 = 45$.

In order to calculate I_1, we need the values of the variable "sex", that is, all the data in the corresponding column. Similarly, I_2 is calculated from all the data for the variable "age". The indicator I_3, however, depends on the two variables "sex" and "age" together. In order to calculate it, we need to know, for every consultation, both the sex and the age of the patient. Thus an indicator depends on one or on several variables as a whole whereas data are given for single units. All of these variables have to be defined for the *same* units, in our example for the consultations recorded above.

We can now formulate the general definition of an indicator:

An indicator is a number that depends on a given set of variables, which are all defined for the same units. It is calculated by making use, for every unit, of the values of all of these variables.

For instance we can derive from the variable "diagnosis" the following three indicators: "Number of consultations during the month of January 2018 leading to the diagnosis 'influenza syndrome' or 'measles' or 'traffic accident', respectively".

In Sect. 1.3 we have looked at of the concept of a unit of a register from the angle of its concrete meaning and practical relevance. We noted that the units of the Register of Consultations of a Commune Health Station are indeed consultations, not persons. The same person can consult the station several times, either for the same complaints or for different ones. In some types of analyses, this distinction between "consultation" and "person" plays no essential role, in others it does; it should always be kept in mind.

11.2 Registers

There are many registers in a health station, policlinic or hospital. Most of them have two basically different functions. Let us resume them briefly before entering into details:

The first function of a register in a health institution is to use the recorded *data* directly in the work of the institution. The second function consists in deriving *indicators* that are partly employed in the institution itself and partly reported to administrative institutions.

In addition, registers can also be used for epidemiologic studies about the link between several variables, usually a risk factor and an outcome variable.

There will be examples of such studies later on, starting with Sect. 11.3.

We are going to look at the first two functions defined above for the various registers in a Commune Health Station. We start with the Register of Consultations. Its first, and most important function is clinical or, more generally, case-management. Entering data such as symptoms and diagnosis into the register instead of only recording them mentally makes it indeed easier for the practising physician or health worker to get a clear idea about the case and to reach a good decision about the treatment. This is particularly true for consultations within a strategy of public health such as ARI or CDD, which use a standardized decision scheme. For example in the strategy CDD described in Sect. 6.4, the diagnosis is based on a few clinical standard symptoms. It consists in a number, namely the degree of dehydration, which is recorded and which determines the treatment.

Additional data such as the date of the consultation and the name and address of the patient are indispensable if there are several consultations for the same case. They are also needed in order to follow up a case. The data "health insurance number" and "payment" are obviously important as well. They are required in the financial management of the Station and belong only indirectly to the subject "epidemiology"of our book; see Sect. 2.1. We shall therefore not treat them here.

The second function of the Register of Consultations of a Commune Health Station is to calculate *indicators*. Some of them concern finances and management but again we are only interested in epidemiologic indicators such as disease frequencies and mortalities. Knowing these indicators is, in the first place, important for the staff of the station itself in order to plan their activities. In the second place, for about 20 infectious diseases and for some types of injuries and poisoning, incidences and mortalities by three age groups (<5, $5–14$, >14) are reported quarterly to the Health Centre of the district to which the commune belongs. These reports form one of the primary-level components of the health information system to be discussed in the following section.

There are many more registers in a Commune Health Station in addition to the one on consultations, for example the general Register of Vaccinations of Children, which concerns essentially the vaccinations in the programme EPI (Expanded Programme on Immunization): Poliomyelitis, diphtheria, pertussis, tetanus, measles and hepatitis B. A unit of this register is a child. The register has, again, two functions. Firstly, for a given child, the data in the corresponding row allow the follow-up of the vaccinations of this child, that is, its vaccination status. Secondly, from the register one calculates, and reports quarterly, the number of vaccinations performed during a given quarter.

The "vaccination coverage" of a "cohort" of children is the principal aspect of judging the quality of vaccination in a commune in accordance with EPI. For example the coverage by measles vaccination of the cohort of all children born in the year 2016 is the proportion of these children who lived through their first year and were vaccinated during that first year of life. A child born in 2016 could have been vaccinated in 2016 or in 2017. Therefore, in order to find the vaccination coverage from the registers of vaccinations, one would have to search the register of 2016 and 2017 for the vaccination data of all children born in the commune in 2016 and only for those. This is rather tedious, especially with paper-based registers or computer-based ones without appropriate software. Of course one also has to know the total number of births in the commune in 2016.

All the other registers of epidemiologic relevance in the Commune Health Station have the same two functions. This is true for the register of pregnancies (antenatal examinations), the register of births and follow-up of the newborn, the one of family planning and finally that of case-management for three particular types of diseases: tuberculosis, malaria and mental diseases. There are in fact too many registers. For example having separate registers of pregnancies and of births plus follow-up of children excludes the calculation of certain indicators that are important for the programme Mother and Child Health (MCH); see Sects. 11.3 and 20.2.

Some health stations in smaller communes maintain a register of families, for instance in the form of card files. Here, a unit is a family of the commune, and data for a given family are recorded on one card. This allows the staff of the station to keep an eye on various aspects of the health within their commune like follow-up of pregnancies and examinations of the newborn, vaccination status, and follow-up of treatments of chronic diseases. It is less practicable in larger communes; there, even a computer-based register of families would still demand much time to handle. Moreover, it is not easy to keep track of migrating families.

Policlinics and hospitals have many more registers than Commune Health Stations but they vary much between them; there is no unique scheme for all Vietnamese hospitals. In most hospitals there exists a register of entries and exits (discharges) of patients which, on the one hand, allows to keep track of individual hospitalized persons and, on the other hand, can be used for calculating indicators of the type "number of patients hospitalized in 2010". Many wards of a hospital have their own register of consultations. Laboratories record their activities in a register whose unit is an examination. It is important to realize that the "data" in such a register are to be understood in a very general sense. For example, in an X-ray department the data for an examination consist of one or several X-ray pictures plus their evaluation by the radiologist.

In larger hospitals, there usually exists a central patient register, which is also called a "master"-register. Its unit is a patient, and for every patient one records here all the places in the various registers of the hospital listed above where this patient appears and where data on his hospitalizations can be found. Thus the master-register provides a link between all registers.

The totality of all registers in a hospital and of links between them is called a "hospital information system".

It is nowadays often carried by suitable computer software but there is no principal difference between a "paper-based" and a "computer-based" hospital information system; the basic ideas are the same. A computer-based hospital information system allows of course to establish links much more rapidly and also permits fast evaluation of the work of the hospital via the calculation of indicators.

11.3   Health Information Systems

Health information systems in Vietnam have already been mentioned briefly in the Sects. 2.1 and 4.5. A general definition might look like this:

A Health Information System (HIS) consists in the regular exchange of indicators and data within or between health institutions following fixed rules.

A hospital information system as sketched in the preceding section is a good example. It handles both data and indicators. Another example is the reporting system for epidemic surveillance described in Sect. 4.5; it concerns mainly data. Registers for particular diseases, for instance the cancer register described in Sect. 22.1, are health information systems as well.

However, when health officials in a country like Vietnam talk about a health information system they usually have in mind exchanges within a large set of health institutions, comprising on the one hand health stations and hospitals where people are being treated and on the other hand administrative entities. In Vietnam they mostly mean routine reports about indicators from *all* Commune Health Stations and *any kind* of hospitals to health administrations on higher levels.

Let us look at the structure of such a system. As before, we will restrict ourselves to indicators of epidemiologic relevance although a health information system is also concerned with matters of health economy and health administration.

In the preceding section we have described the primary-level component of Vietnamese health information systems. It is based on registers in Commune Health Stations and consists of regular reports from there to District Health Centres. At the next higher level, we find, among others, regular reports from the District Health Centres to the Health Department of their province. Their frequency depends on the subject; they may be filed quarterly, bi-annually or annually.

These reports from a District Health Centre to a Health Department are based partly on the indicators that the Commune Health Stations of the district have furnished, and partly on reports to the District Health Centre from other health institutions that exist on the district level: the District Hospital or Policlinic and health facilities concerned with particular problems such as AIDS, malaria, tuberculosis, Mother and Child Health (MCH) and family planning. They concern essentially the same subjects as on the primary level but are partly organized in a different way. They are of course also much more detailed. For example, from the hospitals, incidences and mortalities from 302 different diseases, accidents and other health problems are required separately for the age groups 0–4, 5–14 and ≥ 15.

Reporting from the Province Health Department to the Ministry of Health follows essentially the same lines.

On the whole, the Vietnamese health information system is fairly comprehensive but heavy and complex. It places a heavy burden on those handling it, especially in Commune Health Stations. There are several reasons for this, which it is important to understand. Firstly, in a commune all health activities apart from those by private doctors and healers are concentrated in a single place, namely the health station.

This is no longer the case on the district level where there exist all the institutions listed above. In principle the reports to the District Health Centre described above are meant to satisfy also the information needs of these other district health facilities. Thus the District Health Centre ought to forward the information received rapidly to them. In practice, however, the Commune Health Stations are often still asked to send reports directly to other health institutions on the district level in addition to the reports addressed to the District Health Centre. Many so-called vertical programmes are also requiring separate reports.

Secondly registers and reports are required in an uncoordinated way about many subjects and by ill-designed mechanisms.

Thirdly the aspect of the local use of data and indicators in addition to something that needs to be reported (beginning of Sect. 11.2) is not addressed.

In fact, one can hardly speak of "the" health information system; there exist several ones. In particular, there is the so-called "Health *Management* Information System". It had been designed by WHO for developing countries in order to replace former inefficient systems where they existed or to introduce a system where there was none before. However, in spite of claims to the contrary it is not founded on clear ideas about *what* it should do and *how* it could do it. In particular it does not cover all the information needs described above. Some Vietnamese Commune Health Stations are now even working with both the old system and the Health Information Management System. Also it still requires much unnecessary work by the people who are running or using it.

The most serious aspect of the present disintegrated nature of health information including the Health Management Information System is the existence of several separate registers that all concern the same set of units. In particular, in a Commune Health Station there are several registers concerning Mother and Child Health, namely that of antenatal examinations, of the delivery plus follow-up of the newborn, and of vaccinations within EPI. However, in principle they all have the same units. A unit is simply a child from the moment of its conception until the end of its first year of life. Separating them does not only increase the workload of the staff of the station. It also renders impossible epidemiologic studies of relations between the subjects of these registers, for example a study about the influence of antenatal care on the development of the child during the first year of its life. We shall come back to this problem in Lesson 13 but we note already here the following general, and fundamental, principle:

In any health service, for a given set of units, there shall be at most one register.

There are also technical deficiencies. The layout of the present reporting forms from the Commune Health Stations is not adapted to the structure and layout of the registers on which they are based, which makes calculating indicators tedious. The variables of the register needed for calculating a given indicator should always be clearly identified on the reporting form as well. This is also indispensable for computerizing the process.

Clear rules on the analysis and use of the various types of information handled are lacking. For a given indicator there is never an indication on whether it is only needed and used at the health facility where it had been obtained, or is only meant to be reported to a higher level, or both.

This problem of the "local use" of indicators is also connected with the following question. Should a District Health Centre report to its Province Health Department the incidences and mortalities by important diseases separately for every one of its communes, or only the so-called "aggregated", or "consolidated", indicators, that is the totals for all communes together? The first ones are important for planning and managing health activities on the district level but are hardly ever needed by the province health department. Reporting them routinely makes reporting and handling the information unnecessarily heavy regardless of whether the system works on paper or by a computer network.

Finally a basic problem has risen with the arrival of private physicians on the primary level. They are being licensed by Province Health Departments and are not always required to take part in the health information systems of the Commune Health Stations. Hence there are essential gaps in the reports of for instance the incidence of common diseases treated on the primary level. In this way the figures about such incidences given in Health Statistics Yearbooks or reported to WHO become less reliable.

Regarding the local use of data it has happened that a private physician did not have any data because he did not even keep patient files! When he treated a patient for the second time for the same disease he had forgotten what he had done in the first consultation and the patient, a boy in the case in point, did not remember either not did his mother.

11.4   Practical Work

1. Invent a system for coding the main diagnoses that occur in the register of consultations of a Commune Health Station. This system should satisfy the following criteria:

   - Each diagnosis is represented by a three-letter code such as CUM.
   - These codes are based on the Vietnamese words of the diagnoses and are easy to remember.
   - The system is "compatible" with the 10th Revision of the International Classification of Diseases (ICD-10) in the following sense: each three-letter code corresponds to one or several categories of the ICD-10. Example: The three-letter code for the diagnosis "viral hepatitis" would correspond to the categories B 15–B 19.

2. In a commune to be visited, find the vaccination coverage of the cohort of all children born there in January 2016 for the following vaccinations:

   • Poliomyelitis (Sabin three times).
   • Measles.
   • DTP (three times).
   • Full vaccination in the sense of EPI (without hepatitis B), that is, the seven vaccinations mentioned before together.

   Decide first which parts of which register in the station you need to consult.

Lesson 12
The Origin of Information: Sampling

Sampling is the art of obtaining information on a target population by studying only a suitably chosen subpopulation. The latter is called a sample or a study population. The information includes a description of the error committed by using only a sample. Almost every epidemiologic study involves sampling, but sampling may also be performed regularly within a given information system.

12.1   The Concept of a Sampling Error

Sampling from medical records is a classical technique in medical and epidemiologic research. Let us look at a fictitious example from the pre-computer age. Suppose Dr. Q. wants to find the frequency of a risk factor A among all patients who were treated in a given ward of his hospital during the period 1950–1959. There had been $N = 9850$ such patients, and for every one of them a medical record in the form of a file exists where the presence or absence of A is recorded. Dr. Q. could look through the whole (dust covered) set of files and count the occurrence of A in it. Suppose that he finds it 271 times; this would be the "frequency" he is looking for. The so-called "relative frequency", or "proportion", of A is more instructive; it is equal to

$$\bar{x} = 271 / 9{,}850 = 0.027513 \approx 2.75\%.$$

Going through all the files is time consuming, though, and Dr. Q. might be satisfied with an *estimate* of the unknown proportion $\bar{x}$ by examining only a *sample S_1* of files, for example every tenth file, starting with the first one. If he finds the factor A recorded 25 times in his $n = 985$ extracted files, then the proportion of A in the sample S_1 is equal to

$$\bar{x}_1 = 25 / 985 = 0.025381 \approx 2.54\%.$$

This so-called "sample proportion" $\bar{x}_1$ is Dr. Q's "estimate" of the "population proportion" $\bar{x}$, obtained on the basis of the sample S_1.

© Springer Nature Switzerland AG 2019
K. Krickeberg et al., *Epidemiology*, Statistics for Biology and Health,
https://doi.org/10.1007/978-3-030-16368-6_12

When dealing with $\bar{x}_1$ instead of $\bar{x}$, Dr. Q. commits the "sampling error", or "error" for short, of

$$\bar{x} - \bar{x}_1 = 0.002132.$$

A more informative quantity is the "relative error", that is, the error relative to the quantity to be estimated. It is equal to

$$(\bar{x} - \bar{x}_1)/\bar{x} = 0.077491 \approx 7.7\%.$$

Both the error and the relative error are of course unknown to Dr. Q. The basic idea of modern sampling methods is to obtain, instead of the error in a particular sample, an idea about the error that one can *expect in general* when looking at all possible samples. We are going to make this precise.

Starting the sample with the first file is a rather arbitrary decision. Dr. Q. could as well select one of the numbers 1, ..., 10 at random with the same probability 1/10, using a simple random mechanism such as a roulette wheel, a table of random numbers or the random number programme on his pocket calculator. If, for example, he would get in this way the number 9, his sample, to be called S_9, would consist of the files numbered 9, 19, 29, 39, ..., 9849. The corresponding sample proportion $\bar{x}_9$ would most likely be different from his former estimate $\bar{x}_1$. The sample and therefore the sample proportion now depend on chance. The sample proportion is a "random variable" in the language of probability theory; vaguely speaking a random variable is a number that depends on chance.

In this book we do not assume knowledge of probability theory. For those who ignore the basic concepts of this domain, it suffices to have an intuitive idea of what "on the average" means. A random variable such as the "sample proportion" has an average value, which is called its "mean", or "expected", value.

As said before, Dr. Q. is interested in the *error* committed when he uses his estimate instead of the true but unknown proportion $\bar{x}$. For purely mathematical reasons one usually works with the square of the error instead of the error itself, that is, with $(\bar{x} - \bar{x}_S)^2$ if S is the sample obtained by the random choice above and $\bar{x}_S$ the corresponding sample proportion. Thus the squared error, too, is a random variable since it depends on S. One regards the *mean*, or expected, value of the squared error as the fundamental quantity that describes the "quality" of an estimation procedure like the one above; it is called the "mean square error" and will be denoted by M^2. Having a small mean square error is a desirable feature of an estimation procedure. The quantity $M = \sqrt{M^2}$ is a measure of the *average deviation* of $\bar{x}_S$ from $\bar{x}$ in a slightly generalized sense; it is called its "standard deviation". Again, the "relative" standard deviation, that is, $M/\bar{x}$, provides a better impression of the quality of the estimation.

The mean square error depends on the unknown distribution of the factor A among the files; hence Dr. Q. does not know beforehand how good his estimation procedure is. The basic idea of modern sampling methods takes now the following concrete form:

The *same* sample S that had been selected for estimating the population proportion $\bar{x}$ will also be used for estimating the mean square error M^2.

We shall pursue this idea further in Sect. 12.3.

12.2 Sampling Plans

Let us regard a file as a "unit" and describe the presence or absence of the factor A by a variable defined on these units. We number the files from 1 to $N = 9850$ and we set $x_i = 1$ if A was present for the patient having file no. i and $x_i = 0$ if not. The sequence of these *unknown data* $x_1, \ldots, x_{9,850}$ is then a variable as defined in Sect. 11.1 and $\bar{x}$ is the arithmetic mean of the data.

The quality of the estimation procedure depends on the unknown data. It can be very bad; let us look at our artificial example. Suppose that, for easy management, the nurses who had taken care of the files had always arranged them in groups of 10. Since patients with the factor A required special treatment, they had placed their files within each group at the end. There had never been more than one file with the factor A in a single group of 10. Then the sample proportions $\bar{x}_1, \ldots, \bar{x}_9$ would all be equal to 0, and the relative errors of these estimates of $\bar{x}$ would be equal to 100%! The sample proportion $\bar{x}_{10}$, however, would be equal to $10 \cdot \bar{x}$, which is an even worse estimate; it has the relative error 900%. Finally, the mean square error would be $M^2 = 9 \cdot \bar{x}^2$.

Dr. Q.'s method for taking a sample of files is called a "systematic sampling plan" with the "sampling interval" 10. The reason for its poor performance for the particular data in our artificial example is obvious: the unknown data contain a periodic element whose period is equal to the sampling interval.

For any target set whose units have been arranged in some order we define a systematic sampling plan, with any sampling interval, in a completely analogous fashion. As a practical though vague rule we may then say that such a plan will be appropriate if we can assume the unknown data to behave more or less "completely at random" and in particular without any hidden periodicities.

A systematic sampling plan is easy to execute and often used but, as we have seen, depending on the unknown data it may not always furnish good estimates. Hence the question of using other and better sampling methods arises. We are going to define the concept of a *general* sampling plan for selecting a sample S from a given target set U of "units". These units are also called "observation units" and may be anything, for example communes, hospitals, laboratories, X-ray pictures or, as in Dr. Q.'s problem, medical record files. In many studies they are persons and U is then a population in the usual sense of non-technical language. In sampling theory and practice one often uses the word "population" for *any* target set.

In order to draw a sample from U in practice, one needs a concrete representation of the units. This is called a "sampling frame"; we shall meet many examples later on. For theoretical purposes it is convenient to imagine that the units have been numbered, from 1 to N, say, where N is the "population size". To simplify matters further we shall *identify* these numbers with the corresponding units so that we speak for example about the unit 27 instead of the unit that carries the number 27. Thus, the target set becomes the set of numbers $U = \{1, ..., N\}$ and a sample from U is a subset of U, that is, a set S of different numbers $u_1,..., u_n$ written as

$$S = \left\{u_1,...,u_n\right\}.$$

Each u_i is one of the numbers 1, ..., N and n is the so-called "sample size" and n/N the "sampling fraction". We now define:

A sampling plan is a procedure by which a sample is selected from the target set with a probability given beforehand.

Thus in order to determine a sampling plan, we have to indicate, for every possible sample from U, the probability with which it will be selected. In the systematic sampling plan above with $N = 9850$, each sample of the form

$$S = \left\{v,v+10,v+20,...,v+9{,}840\right\}$$

where v is one of the numbers 1, ..., 10, has the probability 1/10 to be chosen. Its sample size is always equal to 985 and its sampling fraction is 1/10. All other samples have the probability 0 to be selected.

Next, we define the so-called "simple" sampling plan. Let n be a whole number (an "integer") such that $1 \leq n \leq N$; it is going to be the size of every sample to be selected. As every child in the last years of secondary school should know, there exist

$$_N C_n = N\left(N-1\right)\left(N-2\right)...\left(N-n+1\right)/n!$$

samples of size n from a target set U of size N where $n! = 1 \times 2 \times ... \times n$. In the simple sampling plan with sample size n, all of them have, by definition, the same probability to be selected, namely $1/_N C_n$; all samples of a size different from n have probability 0.

In order to "implement" this plan, that is, to actually construct a sample, we could in principle make a list of all the $_N C_n$ samples from U of size n and then select one by a random mechanism of the kind mentioned above (table of random numbers, computer,...). This is, however, rarely practicable since $_N C_n$ is very large even for moderately sized target sets and sample sizes. Another method looks like this: select first a unit u_1 from U, all units having the same probability $1/N$ to be selected; next, select a unit u_2 from the set U from which the unit u_1 has been removed, every unit in this set having the same probability $1/(N-1)$ to be selected; and so on until the sample $S = \{u_1,..., u_n\}$ is complete. This method, too, becomes cumbersome for large N. Moreover, both methods assume that the target set U is given in a concrete and explicit form, which we had called a sampling frame. For example, if we want to select a sample of 9 households from among all households of the hamlet Dong Tam in the commune An Dong, district Quynh Phu, province Thaí Bình by a simple sampling plan, we would first need a list of all households of Dong Tam. Note that, in contrast, Dr. Q. could start implementing his systematic sampling plan without even knowing beforehand how many files there were altogether.

Demographers talk about a "census"; this means taking as a sample the *whole* target population. Formally, this is a simple sampling plan where $n = N$.

The next sampling plan to be discussed is called "Madow's plan". It is applied in a situation where each unit of the target set U has a well-defined "size" or "extension". For example, the units may be the communes of the province of Thaí Bình, and the "size" of a commune may be the number of its inhabitants. It then appears reasonable to attach a higher importance to larger communes than to smaller ones, and this can be achieved by a plan such that, for every commune, the probability that it belongs to the sample chosen is *proportional to its size*. There exist several plans with this property but among them Madow's plan is most frequently used in practical epidemiology. We shall first describe the underlying idea with the help of the example just mentioned and then indicate how to proceed in practice.

We need a sampling frame in the form of a list of the $N = 285$ communes of the province of Thaí Bình and of their number of inhabitants. Denote by h_u the number of inhabitants of the commune no. u, for $u = 1,\ldots, N$. Then $h = h_1 + h_2 + \ldots + h_N$ is the number of inhabitants of the whole province. Next we calculate the sequence of the "cumulated numbers of inhabitants" $h_1, h_1 + h_2, h_1 + h_2 + h_3,\ldots$ and look at the sets of numbers between two successive cumulated numbers:

$$\{1,\ldots,h_1\}$$
$$\{h_1 +1,\ldots,h_1 + h_2\}$$
$$\{h_1 + h_2 +1,\ldots,h_1 + h_2 + h_3\}$$
$$\ldots$$
$$\ldots \tag{12.1}$$
$$\{h_1 +\ldots+ h_{N-1} +1,\ldots,h\}.$$

Recall that for example $\{1, \ldots, h_1\}$ is the set that consists of the numbers 1, 2, $\ldots, h_1$. In sampling theory, sets of this form are called "intervals". Thus, the "length", or "size", of the u-th interval above is equal to the number h_u of inhabitants of the corresponding commune no. u. Therefore, if we wanted to select only a *single* commune with a probability proportional to its size, we could simply chose a number k at random from among the numbers $1,\ldots,h$, each number having the same probability to be chosen, and then select the commune no. u if k falls into the u-th interval.

However, how to select *several* communes at a time, that is, to select an entire sample of given sample size n? The underlying idea is inspired by systematic sampling. We define again a "sampling interval". Essentially, it is the number h of all inhabitants of the province divided by n but since this quotient h/n may not be a whole number, the sampling interval l is defined as the largest whole number less than or equal to h/n, usually written as

$$l = [h/n].$$

In the last step of the construction of the sample S we select a number k at random from this interval, every one of its numbers having the same probability $1/l$ of being selected, and calculate the n numbers

$$k, \ k+l, \ k+2l, ..., \ k+(n-1)l. \qquad (12.2)$$

Every one of them falls into one of the intervals (12.1) above, and S is to consist of the corresponding communes.

In practice, one will use a table with four columns. The first one is the sampling frame and is called "Names of the communes"; thus the table has a row for every commune. The next two columns carry the headings "Number of inhabitants" and "Cumulated number of inhabitants". In the fourth column one writes the numbers (12.2) in the appropriate lines as determined by the third column; this defines the sample. The student should do it in the context of the Practical Work 2, below.

However, two remarks are in order. Firstly, if h/n is not a whole number, the probability of a commune to be included in the sample will in general only be approximately be proportional to its "size". In practice this difference can be neglected.

Secondly, if there exist some communes that are larger than the sampling interval, that is, if

$$l < \max(h_1, ..., h_N),$$

then one of the intervals (12.1) may contain *several* numbers of the sequence (12.2) and we would thus have to include the corresponding commune several times into the sample. We will not enter into the finer mathematical points to deal with this situation. In practice, it will hardly ever happen because taking a sample from a population is only of interest if the sample size n is small compared to the population size N. The sample size n is then all the more small compared to h so that h/n and therefore l will be larger than all commune sizes h_u.

The sampling plans to be presented next take into account a "stratification" of the target set U. We start with an example; several more will come up later. We want to extract a sample from the set U of all hospitals that exist in the region for which the Medical University of Thai Binh is training physicians. Small hospitals including policlinics have a very different structure from medium ones, and large hospitals are again different. Hence it may be reasonable to study separately the three "strata" of which U is composed:

U_1: all small hospitals; U_2: all medium hospitals; U_3: all large hospitals.
Let N_1, N_2 and N_3 be their respective sizes so that $N = N_1 + N_2 + N_3$ is the total number of hospitals.

A "stratified sampling plan" for taking a sample of hospitals looks like this. For every stratum U_j with $j = 1, 2, 3$ we give ourselves a sampling plan. Then we select, *independently* of each other, samples S_1, S_2 and S_3 from U_1, U_2 and U_3, respectively, according to these plans. The final sample S will be these three samples taken together, that is, their union. Thus it will contain small, medium and large hospitals.

Very often, but not always, the plans used in the strata will be simple plans. It is also fairly common to work with fixed sample sizes n_1, n_2 and n_3 in the strata and to make the three sampling fractions n_j/N_j, $j = 1, 2, 3$ approximately the same.

It is obvious how to define a stratified sampling plan for any stratification, that is, for a decomposition of the target set U into J strata $U_1,\ldots, U_J$.

We shall now generalize the concept of a stratified sampling plan, and start again with an example. The target set U is the set of all households of the district of Quynh Phu of the province of Thaí Bình. We number the 38 communes of this district and denote by U_j the set of all households of the commune no. j, for $j = 1, \ldots, 38$. Thus we have stratified U into the strata $U_1,\ldots, U_{38}$. If we want to take a sample from U, we can of course apply a stratified plan, that is, select a sample of households from every commune. We might argue, however, that the various communes of the district are fairly similar and that it may therefore suffice to select a sample of households only from *some* communes, but not from all of them. This leads us to the concept of a "two-stage sampling plan".

A two-stage sampling plan is based on a stratification $U_1 ,\ldots, U_J$ of the target set U. It is determined by a sampling plan P for taking *first* a sample from the set of strata $\{U_1 ,\ldots, U_J\}$ and then, for each stratum U_j with $j = 1, \ldots, J$, a sampling plan P_j for taking a sample from this stratum.

In order to implement the plan, we do the following. At the first stage, we select a sample of strata by using the plan P. At the second stage, we employ the plans P_j for selecting, independently of each other, a sample from each of the strata that were selected at the first stage. The final sample is their union.

We shall now single out three particular types of two-stage sampling plans. Firstly, we know already stratified sampling plans. They are two-stage plans where, at the first stage, we select *all* strata. In other words, **P** is a census.

In the two-stage plans of the second type to be defined it is, on the contrary, the plans P_j *within* the strata by which we select *all* elements. This means that at the first stage, we draw a sample of strata and the final sample is just the union of these. Thus, the strata drawn are included in the final sample as a whole and they are therefore called "clusters"; the plan is called "cluster sampling". For example, suppose we want to investigate the state of malnutrition of all children aged under 5 in a commune; this is the target population. A stratum consists of all children under 5 in the same family, or household. We first select, by some plan, a sample of households; these are the clusters. Then we investigate *all* children under 5 in the selected households.

The third particular type of two-stage sampling plans is defined by the fact that the plan **P** at the first stage, that is, for selecting strata, is a Madow plan. The plans P_j for selecting, at the second stage, samples from the strata chosen at the first stage may be anything, depending on the situation. For example, if the observation units are the households and the strata are the hamlets of a given commune, we may proceed as follows. At the first stage we select some hamlets by Madow's plan. At the second stage we obtain, for these selected hamlets, sampling frames in the form of lists of their households and we employ simple random sampling. For the reason given in the following section, it is advantageous to use the same sample size in all strata, for example to choose 11 households from each hamlet selected by Madow's plan.

There is no special term to denote this type of two-stage sampling plan. In the particular case of 30 strata to be selected at the first stage, WHO uses the name "30-cluster plan" although it is not a cluster sampling plan according to the generally accepted statistical terminology as defined above.

12.3   Indicators and Sample Statistics

The traditional purpose of sampling has been to estimate the mean, or average, value of a variable X defined on the observation units; it is called the "population mean". For example let the target set consist of all households in the district of Quynh Phu. The variable X is "health care expenditure in the year 2016". We number the households from 1 to N and denote by x_u the expenditure for health of the household no. u during the year 2016. Then the population mean is the "*average* health care expenditure per household in Quynh Phu during 2016*", that is,

$$\bar{x} = \left(1 / N\right)(x_1 + x_2 + \ldots + x_N).$$

A population mean is an indicator as defined in Sect. 11.1. We have noted in the beginning of the preceding section that a population proportion is a particular case of a population mean; it results if each value x_u is equal to 0 or 1. In the sequel we shall also look at other "population indicators". They are sometimes called population "parameters" but the term parameter in this sense should be avoided because it may lead to confusion.

Now we pass from population indicators to sample indicators. An indicator on a sample S, which can be calculated from the "known data" x_u for all units u of S, regarded as depending on S, is also called a "sample statistic". The "sample mean" $\bar{x}_S$ of X, that is, the sum of the data for the units in the sample S divided by the sample size, is a particular case. Note that sample indicators are *not* parameters in the usual statistical terminology.

In many investigations one is also interested in other indicators, not only in means; we will look at examples below. There again, one frequently uses the following heuristic principle that had already guided us in Sect. 12.1:

In the first place envisage estimating a population indicator by the corresponding sample indicator.

This is, however, not always the best strategy. Depending on the underlying sampling plan even the sample mean may not be the most appropriate estimator of the population mean. For example for the two-stage sampling plans described above where the first stage plans were Madow's, we had recommended to use, at the second stage, sampling plans with the same sample size in all strata selected. In that case, the sample mean as an estimator of the population mean is "unbiased". This property, which we will not treat here, is sometimes considered desirable. If different sample sizes are used in the strata, the sample mean may be a "biased" estimator of the population mean.

We shall now return to the fundamental question with which we had started the present lesson, namely that of the error committed "in general" when estimating a population mean $\bar{x}$ by the sample mean $\bar{x}_S$. As we did in Sect. 12.1 we shall consider the squared error $(\bar{x} - \bar{x}_S)^2$ for the randomly selected sample S and define the mean square error M^2 as its mean, or "expected", value. This is a good measure of the quality of the underlying sampling plan. It is of course unknown to the investigator. However, in order to get an idea of the mean square error, he may apply the heuristic principle stated above and *estimate* M^2 by a corresponding sample indicator based on the same sample.

For a simple sampling plan, this idea leads to the following result. First we define the so-called "sample variance" s_S^2 for a sample S: take the sum of all numbers $(x_u - \bar{x}_S)^2$ for all units u in S and divide it by $n - 1$. Then we have the following basic result, which we formulate in the not altogether precise form in which it is being applied:

$$s_S^2(1 - n/N)/n \text{ is a "useful" estimate of } M^2.$$

In most applications the sample fraction n/N is small and can be neglected compared with the term 1. Then this estimate of the mean square error M^2 takes the form s_S^2/n.

The sample variance, like the sample mean, is an example of a sample statistic. The usual statistical software provides both the sample mean $\bar{x}_S$ and the sample variance s_S^2 upon entry of the data x_u for all u in the sample S.

We shall learn in Lesson 14 how to derive from the mean square error M^2 other ways of describing errors committed by sampling. Any report on the results of a sample survey should contain a description of the methods employed.

Finally, recall that the preceding discussion of the estimation of the mean square error holds for a simple sampling plan. We cannot enter here into the problem of estimating it for other plans, for example for two-stage plans. In practice one often argues that the methods that are valid for a simple sampling plan can also be used "approximately" for other plans, for example a systematic or a Madow plan.

12.4   Choice of a Sampling Plan

When conducting a sample survey, the investigator evaluates the information contained in his sample by calculating for example a sample mean and a sample variance and he draws conclusions from them. He does this at the end of the study, just before writing his report. At the beginning, given his research question, he has to reach a decision about the "sampling strategy", which consists of the sampling plan and appropriate estimators. His first step is, as always, a precise description of the target population. Next, he has to define the variables whose means he wants to estimate. In practice one almost always tries to estimate, by the same sampling plan, the mean of not only one but of several variables. This poses statistical problems that are unfortunately often neglected. Here, we will restrict ourselves to the estimation of a single population mean by the corresponding sample mean.

Given the objectives, the choice of a sampling plan is determined by two elements:
- **Feasibility including cost.**
- **The sampling error.**

The first element is composed of things such as the structure of the target set, for example a given natural stratification or administrative structure; the existence or possible construction of sampling frames; finances and collaborators; ways to reach the units of a sample such as hamlets or households and to record the information on them; controlling mistakes when recording information (the so-called "non-sampling errors"); etc. We shall take up these technical matters in Lesson 27.

Regarding the second element, the investigator usually has a more or less precise idea of the order of magnitude of the sampling errors that he still considers admissible. The sampling error does not only depend on the sampling plan but also on the variable whose mean is to be estimated, that is, on the unknown data. Very often, however, before starting his study, the investigator has already some *partial* knowledge about the unknown data. It is then reasonable to try to take this "a priori knowledge" into account when choosing a sampling plan. For example, if Dr. Q. is convinced that his files are arranged in a "completely random" order, he decides to use a systematic sampling plan.

Let us present another application of the same idea. Suppose that we are confronted with a stratification of the target set and that we have only two alternatives: a stratified or a cluster sampling plan. For example the units may be the households of the district of Quynh Phu and each stratum may consist of all households of one of the 38 communes of that district. We had already argued that, if all communes look more or less alike, a sample of strata instead of all strata would be sufficient at the first sampling stage. By including these selected strata *as a whole* in the final sample in order to get a faithful picture of the situation *within* each stratum, we would have a cluster sampling plan. More generally, we will opt for a cluster plan if we suspect that the variation of the data *between* the strata is relatively small whereas the data may fluctuate a lot *within* the strata. In contrast to that, a stratified plan would be called for if we have reasons to believe that there is much variation of data *between* the strata but fairly little *within* them.

Another way to obtain some partial knowledge before embarking on a large sample survey is to make first a "pilot survey" with a small sample where the various components of the planned survey are tried out.

Finally, we can often exploit the results of other sample surveys that had been done before in similar situations. In all these situations we are guided by the same fundamental principle of statistics:

Always try to use any "a priori" information you may already have.

We shall apply this principle again in the following section to the problem of choosing a sample size.

In the practice of survey sampling many investigators do unfortunately not know the basic ideas of sampling theory sufficiently well. In particular, the so-called 30-cluster plan has been used in Vietnam in situations where other plans would have provided more precise results at much less cost and less work.

Let us conclude by adding a few general remarks. For the sake of concreteness we have restricted ourselves to the estimation of a single population mean but we have mentioned that in practice a sample survey usually deals with several variables at a time. Now, most epidemiologic studies as treated in the Lessons 16–20 also make use of appropriate samples. Nevertheless there is a basic difference between normal sample surveys and epidemiologic studies:

In sample surveys, "target" variables are analyzed *separately* whereas the purpose of epidemiologic studies is to investigate *relations* between several variables, for example between a risk factor and an outcome variable.

Sample surveys are usually planned ad hoc to deal with a particular research question. However, they can also take place regularly and routinely, in particular in the framework of a surveillance system. Serosurveillance in certain countries is a prominent example. As remarked in Sect. 4.5, a network of sentinel sites practices sample surveys routinely.

Sample surveys are often expensive. Nevertheless many superfluous surveys have been executed in Vietnam in situations where the information sought for either already existed from other surveys or could have easily been extracted from registers and health information systems. The reason usually is the lack of coordination between several organizations that are active in the health sector.

Sometimes it also turns out that the indicators one wants to obtain are not really needed with high precision and that simplified methods such as the so-called "rapid assessments" suffice.

12.5   Choice of a Sample Size

This is a particular aspect of choosing a sampling plan. We shall treat it only for a simple plan. As remarked at the end of Sect. 12.3, one often applies the results also to other plans such as a systematic or a Madow plan. This may be justified for certain types of variables on the target population but it is frequently being done out of pure ignorance.

First we define the "population variance" s^2 of the given variable X in complete analogy to the sample variance s_S^2 defined in Sect. 12.3. It is the sum of all $(x_i - \overline{x})^2$, divided by $N - 1$. Then it can be shown that in the case of a small sampling fraction n/N, the mean square error M^2 is approximately equal to s^2/n, in a formula:

$$M^2 \approx s^2/n \tag{12.3}$$

The reader should establish the link with the statement made in Sect. 12.3 that s_s^2/n is a useful *estimate* of M^2. This referred to the situation *at the end* of the sample survey where the sample S is already selected. The components of the formula (12.3), however, are independent of a particular sample and we are going to use it precisely to treat the following problem to be solved *before* the survey: how large should the sample size n be in order to provide a mean square error M^2 of a given size that the investigator considers desirable? The relation (12.3) gives immediately a first solution:

$$n \approx s^2 / M^2 \tag{12.4}$$

This looks natural since it implies that one needs a large sample size n whenever the fluctuation of the data in the target population as expressed by s^2 is large or the desired mean square error M^2 is small.

Of course the investigator does not know the population variance s^2 but it often happens that he or she has at least a vague preliminary idea of its order of magnitude, in most cases from a pilot survey or from similar studies already made elsewhere. For example, if she feels sure that s^2 cannot be larger than 100, then (12.4) tells her that her sample size n need not be larger than $100/M^2$. In this way she has applied the principle of using a priori information.

We now pursue this idea further in the particular case of sampling for proportions where the variable X on the target population takes only the values 0 and 1. Our example of Dr. Q.'s files was of this type. We may also think of the following example: the target population is the entire adult population of the province of Thaí Bình, and $x_i = 1$ if and only if the diastolic blood pressure of the inhabitant no. i on the morning of the third February 2016 was higher than 80 mmHg. Then $p = \overline{x}$ is the proportion of these people in Thaí Bình. It can be proved that the population variance is equal to

$$s^2 = p(1-p)N/(N-1)$$

hence for large N we have

$$s^2 \approx p(1-p)$$

so that the relation (12.4) implies

$$n \approx p(1-p)/M^2 \tag{12.5}$$

where p is the unknown proportion that we want to estimate.

If we do not know anything about p, we can use the inequality $p(1-p) \leq 1/4$ that is valid for every p between 0 and 1. This means that even in the worst case a sample size of $n \approx 1/(4\,M^2)$ will be sufficient. However, in practice we can usually do much better because we may already have some idea about the magnitude of p from a pilot survey or another study. Then we assume that p is close to a known quantity $\tilde{p}$ and work with the sample size n obtained from (12.5) by replacing p by $\tilde{p}$, that is,

$$n \approx \tilde{p}(1 - \tilde{p}) / M^2 \tag{12.6}$$

Finally, which mean square error M^2 should we strive for? In Sect. 12.1 we had already remarked that usually *relative* errors are much more informative when estimating proportions. Thus we should like to obtain that the relative mean square error M^2/p^2 be equal to a given number ε^2. In other words the relative standard deviation M/p of the estimated value from the real proportion should be a given number ε. This amounts to $M^2 = \varepsilon^2 p^2$. Replacing again the unknown p by $\tilde{p}$, we get from (12.6) the desired sample size.

$$n \approx \frac{1 - \tilde{p}}{\tilde{p}} \frac{1}{\varepsilon^2} \tag{12.7}$$

In many studies we know already that p is fairly small; a frequent example is the incidence rate of a rare disease, that is, the incidence divided by the population number (see Sect. 15.1). Then we may neglect the term $\tilde{p}$ in the difference $1 - \tilde{p}$ and (12.7) finally takes the simple form.

$$n \approx \frac{1}{\tilde{p}} \frac{1}{\varepsilon^2} \tag{12.8}$$

This shows that a large sample size is required not only for a small relative mean square error ε^2 but also for a small proportion p. For example, if the investigator would like to obtain a relative standard deviation of $\varepsilon = 0.05 = 5\%$ and he thinks that p might be close to $\tilde{p} = 0.01 = 1\%$, he needs a sample size of 39,600. Such a sample survey would be very expensive!

12.6   Practical Work

1. Select a sample of size 3 from the set $\{1, 2, \ldots, 10\}$ by a simple sampling plan.
2. Select a sample of 5 hamlets from the set of all hamlets of a commune of your choice by Madow's plan, the "size" of a hamlet being the number of its households.
3. Organize and implement a sample survey in order to estimate the mean number of missing and the mean number of decayed and unfilled teeth among children aged 10–14 in a commune. Give reasons for the choice of your sampling plan, discuss the various problems, and include estimates of the mean square errors based on the assumption that your sampling plan was a simple one (even when it was not!).

Lesson 13
Descriptive Data Analysis and Statistics

This lesson presents the basic elements of the statistical analysis of data, independently of their origin. In its last section, some first indications are given on where and how such an analysis is needed in epidemiology.

13.1 Data

The two previous lessons have shown us the ways in which most data arise in Public Health. The first way passes through systematic recording in registers. There, data are usually measured and recorded for *all* units of the target population, for example for all consultations in the outpatient ward of the District Hospital of the district of Quynh Phu during the month of January 2018. The second way leads through sampling. Having drawn a sample of units from a given target population we are dealing with "sample data". They are data that were measured and recorded *only* for the units in the sample, that is, in the study population. There also exist the unknown "population data" in the target population.

Whatever the origin of the data may be, we are confronted with a sequence of units, which are already numbered or which we can number. In the present lesson we shall illustrate all concepts and methods with the help of the following example, which is of the type "data from registers". The units are $n = 27$ consultations for cardio-vascular diseases of outpatients in the district hospital of Quynh Phu. We shall meet again some concepts and methods that have already appeared in previous lessons.

In Sect. 11.1 we had defined the concepts "variable" and "indicator." A variable assigns a number to every unit; these numbers are the data with which we are dealing. An indicator is calculated from the entirety of data. Let us look at some variables in the context of our example.

The first variable, to be denoted by Z, is the "sex" of the patient, represented by $z_i = 0$ if the patient in the consultation no. i is male and $z_i = 1$ if this patient is female. This is a so-called "binary" variable as it takes only the two values 0 and 1. Interesting indicators are the sum of all z_i, which is the total number of female

© Springer Nature Switzerland AG 2019
K. Krickeberg et al., *Epidemiology*, Statistics for Biology and Health,
https://doi.org/10.1007/978-3-030-16368-6_13

patients, and their mean $\bar{z}$, which is equal to the proportion of values 1 among all data, that is the number of female patients divided by 27; recall that this is also called their "relative" frequency. Suppose the data $z_1, z_2, ..., z_{27}$ are given by

$$Z: 0\ 0\ 0\ 1\ 0\ 1\ 1\ 1\ 1\ 0\ 1\ 1\ 1\ 1\ 0\ 1\ 0\ 0\ 1\ 1\ 0\ 1\ 0\ 1\ 1\ 0\ 0$$

Each value is to be counted as often as it appears so that we have indeed 27 data altogether. Hence there had been 15 female and 12 male patients. The proportion of female patients was, up to four decimals,

$$\bar{z} = 15 / 27 = 0.5556$$

The second variable will be the "age" X of the patient, expressed in whole years. An example of data $x_1, x_2, ..., x_{27}$:

$$X: 39;\ 84;\ 28;\ 64;\ 35;\ 49;\ 36;\ 75;\ 73;\ 22;\ 28;\ 36;\ 49;\ 64;\ 93;$$
$$89;\ 34;\ 30;\ 77;\ 39;\ 32;\ 86;\ 38;\ 31;\ 95;\ 39;\ 77$$

Again, multiple values such as 28, 36, 39,... are counted as often as they appear. The average, or mean, age of the 27 patients is the so-called "mean" of X, written $\bar{x}$, namely the arithmetic mean $\bar{x} = (x_1 + x_2 + ... + x_{27})/27 = 53.4074$.

Both Z and X are "discrete" variables. By this we mean that there exists, *before* we obtain and record the data, a well-defined finite set of *possible* values for them. In the case of Z, the possible values are 0 and 1; in the case of X, they are 0, 1, 2, ... up to the highest age that is imaginable in the district of Quynh Phu, perhaps 113?

Our third variable will be the diastolic blood pressure measured in mmHg. It is a "continuous" variable Y where in principle all values within a certain range are possible but each of them only with probability 0 (we will not discuss this further). An example of data $y_1, y_2, ..., y_{27}$ where we have, however, rounded the values to entire millimetres:

$$Y: 64;\ 43;\ 76;\ 70;\ 100;\ 109;\ 86;\ 49;\ 83;\ 57;\ 70;\ 60;\ 90;\ 84;\ 87;$$
$$107;\ 73;\ 77;\ 75;\ 61;\ 29;\ 99;\ 29;\ 73;\ 74;\ 83;\ 81$$

The concept of continuous data is useful for statistical theory but in practice they do of course not exist since when measuring and performing calculations we are always dealing with rounded values. The mean of Y, rounded again to the next integer, is equal to $\bar{y} = 74$.

The possible values of the variables X and Y are numbers that are *ordered* by the natural order of numbers and this order has a concrete and relevant meaning. Indeed for any two patients, it is meaningful to state which of the two is older or has a higher diastolic blood pressure unless they happen to have the same age or blood pressure. Variables of this type are called "ordinal".

By contrast, the variable Z is not considered ordinal because the values 0 and 1 that we have chosen rather arbitrarily to represent the two sexes have no intrinsic meaning. Instead, Z is an example of a so-called "categorical" variable where we are given beforehand a set of "categories" of units and the value of the variable for a given unit tells us to which category the unit belongs. In the case of Z there are only two categories "males" and "females". An example with many categories would be "ethnicity", which is also recorded in many registers of consultations. There we have the categories Viet (Kinh), Muong, Cham, Nùng, Ê-dê, Gia-rai, Hoa, Hmông, Kho-me, Tày, Thái and many others.

A categorical variable is of course always discrete. The statistical analysis of categorical variables is in many respects quite different from that of ordinal ones as we shall see below in Sect. 13.4.

13.2 Descriptive Statistical Analysis of One Variable

The first step of any statistical analysis ought to consist in simply looking at the data. Let us start with ordinal data where their magnitude plays a role. In the series X of ages of patients given above we note, for example, that the lowest value is 22 years, which is not astonishing since these patients are consulting for cardio-vascular problems that are rare among children. However, 14 patients, that is, more than half of them, are aged under 40; thus such problems may emerge relatively early in life. Regarding the series of the data for the diastolic blood pressure, there are four very low values, namely 43, 49, 29 and again 29; they may be due to a shock syndrome. Some values are very high.

More generally we shall be interested in the "frequency" of data within a certain range of size. To this end let us arrange them according to their size; a computer can do this quickly. For X, we get the sequence

$$X_0 : 22; 28; 28; 30; 31; 32; 34; 35; 36; 36; 38; 39; 39; 39; 49;$$
$$49; 64; 64; 73; 75; 77; 77; 84; 86; 89; 93; 95$$

For Y, we obtain

$$Y_0 : 29; 29; 43; 49; 57; 60; 61; 64; 70; 70; 73; 73; 74; 75; 76;$$
$$77; 81; 83; 83; 84; 86; 87; 90; 99; 100; 107; 109$$

Data are real numbers. As usual we shall call the set of all real numbers the "real line". By the "distribution" of a variable we mean, intuitively speaking, the distribution of the data over the various parts of the real line. In principle we can describe it by indicating, for every value, the frequency with which this value is taken. For example, the variable Z takes the value 0 altogether 12 times and the value 1 is taken 15 times; no other value is taken. All interesting information that enters into the statistical evaluation of the data can be derived from these two frequencies.

This type of description of a distribution is practical for any discrete variable that does not take too many values, in particular for categorical variables with not too many categories. In its graphical form, which is called its "histogram" it conveys a vivid visual impression of the distribution of the data. The histogram consists in "batons" that are erected over the values. Over each value, a vertical baton is placed whose length is proportional to the frequency with which the value is taken; see Practical Work 1, below.

If the variable takes too many values, most or all values are taken with low frequencies and the resulting histogram does not give a clear picture of the essential aspects of the distribution. For example, X takes the value 39 three times, the values 28, 36, 49, 64 and 77 twice and all other values with the frequency 1 or 0. Similarly, Y takes the values 29, 70, 73 and 83 twice and all other values once or never. In such a case it is preferable to "group" the possible values in an appropriate way. The choice of the groups always requires some thinking. For the variable X, that is "age", we may settle for the eight groups

$$20 - 29, 30 - 39, 40 - 49, 50 - 59, 60 - 69, 70 - 79, 80 - 89, 90 - 99$$

The frequencies of values in these groups are easy to obtain from X_0, above:

$$3, 11, 2, 0, 2, 4, 3, 2$$

Their sum is of course equal to 27. The histogram of X for these age groups is also to be made by the reader; see Practical Work 2. It is constructed by drawing, over each age group represented on the real line, a rectangle whose height is proportional to the frequency of data in this group. Before doing it, one should think about choosing appropriate scales on the two axes. An essential trait of the distribution becomes now visible: the high number of patients aged 30–39. One might speculate that this is due to early over-work but also search for other explanations.

For the diastolic blood pressure Y, we shall work with groups defined by intervals of the length of 15 mmHg in order to avoid a high number of narrow groups, which would lead to mostly low frequencies. Thus we use the six groups:

$$25 - 39, 40 - 54, 55 - 69, 70 - 84, 85 - 99, 100 - 114$$

The corresponding frequencies are

$$2, 2, 4, 12, 4, 3$$

Again, the reader should draw the histogram himself.

It is important to realize that we cannot reconstruct the original distribution from these frequencies or histograms because the latter do not give the data exactly. Calculations of indicators based on grouped data are only approximations to the corresponding exact indicators. To illustrate this, we calculate approximate means $\bar{x}_g$ and $\bar{y}_g$ of X and Y by replacing each exact value by a "mid-point" of the group into which it has fallen. This gives us:

$$\bar{x}_g = \frac{1}{27}\left(3{\cdot}25 + 11{\cdot}35 + 2{\cdot}45 + 0{\cdot}55 + 2{\cdot}65 + 4{\cdot}75 + 3{\cdot}85 + 2{\cdot}95\right) = 52.7778$$

to be compared with $\bar{x} = 53.4074$, and

$$\bar{y}_g = \frac{1}{27}\left(2{\cdot}32 + 2{\cdot}47 + 4{\cdot}62 + 12{\cdot}77 + 4{\cdot}92 + 3{\cdot}107\right) = 74.778 \approx 75$$

to be compared with $\bar{y} = 74$.

Histograms provide a vivid picture of the distribution of a variable of any type. For *ordinal* variables, another kind of description is often more practical. For a given real number ξ we may ask the following question: which proportion of the data is smaller than ξ? By indicating this proportion for every ξ we obtain the so-called "distribution function" of the variable. We shall not pursue this further but ask the opposite question instead, which is of more practical interest: for a given proportion α with $0 < \alpha < 1$, or in other words for a given percentage $\alpha \cdot 100\%$, how do we have to choose ξ such that the percentage of data below ξ is equal to $\alpha \cdot 100\%$? Such a number ξ will be called an "$\alpha{\cdot}100$-percentile" of the variable.

An $\alpha{\cdot}100$-percentile does not exist for every α. For example if $n = 27$, it makes no sense to speak of 5% of the data since 5% of 27 is 1.35 and this is not a whole number. One can still define an $\alpha{\cdot}100$-percentile in the general case while retaining the essential features of the idea of a percentile but this definition is complicated and would be of little practical value for us. Hence we shall do it only in the particular case $\alpha = 1/2$ in order to obtain a "median" of the data, that is, a 50-percentile. The intuitive idea of a median is that half of the data are smaller and half of them are larger than the median. To give a precise definition let us look first at the case of the total number n of units being odd as in our examples where $n = 27$. Then there exists one and only one number $\check{x}$ such that the percentage of data smaller than $\check{x}$ and the percentage of data larger than $\check{x}$ are both less than 50%. This number $\check{x}$ is called the median; it is itself one of the data. For example to find the median $\check{x}$ and $\check{y}$ of the variables X and Y we use the series X_0 and Y_0 of the data arranged in increasing order and get immediately

$$\check{x} = 39 \text{ and } \check{y} = 75$$

In the case of an even number n of data, the precise definition of the median is more involved but the intuitive idea remains the same.

A median is a "central value" of the distribution of the variable; it provides insight into the position of the centre of the data in some sense. We are also interested in a description of the "extension" of the data. First we can simply write down the smallest and the largest value of the data. For X and Y we find

$$x_{\min} = 22, \ x_{\max} = 95 \text{ and } y_{\min} = 29, \ y_{\max} = 109$$

All data are situated between these limits. Next, we want to indicate a region around the centre where *most* of the data are concentrated. This idea, too, can be made precise with the help of percentiles. For example we may consider somewhat arbitrarily that the 5% smallest and the 5% largest data are "far from the centre"; they are, essentially, the data that are smaller than a 5-percentile or larger than a

95-percentile, respectively. Since 5% of 27 is 1.35, only the values 22 and 95 of the variable X would be considered as far from the centre, and for Y it would be the values 29 and 109. Generally speaking, the size of the central region in this sense, namely the length of the interval from a 5- to a 95-percentile, is considered an indicator of the fluctuation of the data. "References values" for laboratory measures, for example of cholesterol in a blood sample, are an important application; any value outside the central interval is regarded as not normal. See also Sect. 19.1.

We obtain the indicators named "percentiles" by *ordering* and *counting* data. Next, let us look at some indicators that are got by *calculating*. We have already calculated the mean of the data in our examples. The mean, too, plays the role of a central value of a distribution. It can be quite different from the median. For X, we had found $\hat{x} = 39$ whereas $\bar{x} = 53$ when rounded to the nearest integer. For Y, however, the median $\hat{y} = 75$ is close to the mean $\bar{y} = 74$. The reason is pretty obvious from the histograms. The distribution of X is very asymmetric around the centre with a high frequency of data in the "young" age group 30–39, which results in a relatively low median whereas the few large data in the age groups over 60 contribute to a larger mean. The distribution of Y is, on the contrary, fairly symmetric, which entails that its median and mean are close to each other.

In a similar vein, the median m of a variable does not change if, for example, the data larger than m are altered while remaining larger than m. Even if we replace some data to the right of m by others that are extremely large, so-called "outliers", the median will remain the same whereas the mean will of course also become very large. In any concrete situation one needs to decide whether the median or the mean provides more appropriate insight about the centre of the distribution.

We also define an indicator which, like 5- and 95-percentiles, is meant to describe some kind of fluctuation of the data but must be calculated. We have already met it in the different context of the preceding lesson; it is called the "variance". Let X be again an *ordinal* variable. We are interested in the deviation of the data x_i from their mean $\bar{x}$. For mathematical reasons we operate with the *squared* deviations $\left(x_i - \bar{x}\right)^2$. The number

$$s^2 = \frac{1}{n-1}\left(\left(x_1 - \bar{x}\right)^2 + \left(x_2 - \bar{x}\right)^2 + \ldots + \left(x_n - \bar{x}\right)^2\right)$$

is essentially the mean of the squared deviations except that, again for mathematical reasons, we have used the denominator $n - 1$ instead of n. If n is not too small, this amounts approximately to the same. The indicator s^2 is the "variance" of the data x_i, that is of the variable X, and the positive square root $s = \sqrt{s^2}$ is its "standard deviation". The standard deviation is the average deviation $|x_i - \bar{x}|$ of the data x_i from their mean $\bar{x}$ where "average" is to be understood not in the ordinary sense as an arithmetic mean but as a slightly modified so-called quadratic mean. Thus a glance at s gives us a rapid impression of the size of the fluctuation of the data.

For the variables X and Y in the preceding section we obtain upon rounding

$$s_x^2 = 567.56, \; s_x = 23.82; \; s_y^2 = 420.38, \; s_y = 20.50$$

Approximate calculations with grouped data are analogous to those presented above for the calculation of a mean.

In Sects. 12.2 and 13.1 we have met *binary* variables, which take only the values 0 and 1. In Sect. 12.2 the value 1 meant "presence of the risk factor A" and in Sect. 13.1 it meant "female". In this case $p = \bar{x}$ is the relative frequency, or proportion, of the value 1 and it is easy to prove that

$$s^2 = \frac{n}{n-1} p(1-p)$$

hence approximately for large n:

$$s^2 \approx p(1-p)$$

Let us stress the obvious:

The indicators "percentile", "median", "mean", "variance", and "standard deviation" are of no interest for categorical variables.

For a binary variable, they are meaningful because we use the particular representation of the two categories by the numbers 0 and 1.

13.3   Descriptive Statistics of Two Ordinal Variables: Correlation, Linear Regression

Up to now we have analyzed variables such as X, Y and Z separately. As remarked in Sect. 12.4 this is what one does in the analysis of several variables which had been obtained in sample surveys. However, the majority of interesting questions in modern statistics, and in particular in epidemiology, are concerned with *relations* between variables. This is inherent in the very definition of epidemiology as the statistical description of relations between factors and outcome variables. In the present lesson we shall only deal with very simple and basic methods of classical statistics. Issues that are specific to epidemiology will be treated in Lessons 15–21.

Let us look at two ordinal variables, for example the variables X and Y of Sect. 13.1. For the patient no. i we have two data, his age x_i and his diastolic blood pressure y_i. We represent them by the point (x_i, y_i) in the xy-plane; this point has the abscissa x_i and the ordinate y_i. When doing it for all patients we obtain 27 points, which form what is called the "data cloud"; see Practical Work 3.

At first sight these data points seem to be fairly irregularly distributed but a closer visual inspection reveals that there seems to be a tendency for older patients to have also higher diastolic blood pressure. We are going to describe this phenomenon in a quantitative way in terms of an indicator. Its definition is founded on the following idea. If such a tendency exists, the deviations from the mean for the two variables, that is, the differences $x_i - \bar{x}$ and $y_i - \bar{y}$ for $i = 1, \ldots, 27$ should in general point into the same direction and in particular should be either both positive or both negative, which would result in positive products $(x_i - \bar{x})(y_i - \bar{y})$. On the contrary, negative products of this type indicate opposite deviations. This makes us consider the arithmetic mean of these products, adjusted as in Sect. 12.3 and 13.2 by dividing not by n but by $n - 1$, namely

$$s_{xy} = \frac{1}{n-1}\left((x_1 - \bar{x})(y_1 - \bar{y}) + (x_2 - \bar{x})(y_2 - \bar{y}) + \ldots + (x_n - \bar{x})(y_n - \bar{y})\right)$$

For two identical variables we obtain of course the variance defined above, that is $s_{xx} = s_x^2$.

The indicator s_{xy} is called the "covariance" of X and Y. It suffers from a drawback: it depends on the scale on which X and Y are measured. For example, if we express the age of a patient not in years but in months, the covariance becomes 12 times larger except for a small correction due to rounding. It is therefore practical to divide s_{xy} by the standard deviations of X and Y in order to obtain an indicator that is independent of the scales on the x- and y-axis. The indicator obtained in this way, namely

$$\rho_{xy} = \frac{s_{xy}}{s_x s_y}$$

is the "correlation coefficient" of X and Y.

We may look upon the correlation coefficient ρ_{xy} as a measure of a "linear" dependence between X and Y. Let us try to make this precise. Firstly, it can be shown that

$$-1 \leq \rho_{xy} \leq 1.$$

Next, $\rho_{xy} = 1$ if and only if the variable Y is a "linearly increasing" function of X, that is it has the form

$$y_i = a + bx_i \text{ for every } i = 1,\ldots,n \tag{13.1}$$

where a and b are constants and b is positive. Geometrically speaking this means that the entire data cloud is situated on the line in the xy-plane given by the equation

$$y = a + bx \tag{13.2}$$

with "intercept" a and a positive "slope" b. Analogously, $\rho_{xy} = -1$ if and only if an equation of the form (13.1) holds for all i where the slope b is negative.

If $-1 < \rho_{xy} < 0$ or $0 < \rho_{xy} < 1$, we consider that there exists only a *partial* linear dependence between X and Y, which is negative or positive, respectively. Finally, if $\rho_{xy} = 0$, we say that X and Y are "uncorrelated".

With the variables in our example we have $\rho_{xy} = 0.2512$. Thus there is indeed a partial, although small, positive linear dependence between them; within the consultations in question older patients tend to have slightly higher diastolic blood pressure.

When using ρ_{xy} as a measure of such a dependence we do not distinguish between "X depends on Y" and "Y depends on X" because $s_{xy} = s_{yx}$ and therefore $\rho_{xy} = \rho_{yx}$. However, as we have recalled in the beginning of this section, in epidemiology we are interested in describing how an "outcome variable" depends on "factors". In the present context we put the problem like this: to describe how the outcome variable "diastolic blood pressure" Y depends on the factor "age" X. It is then customary to call X the "independent" and Y the "dependent" variable.

There are several ways to tackle this problem of dependence, each of them being tied to what is called a statistical "model". The linear regression model is the oldest. In this model we consider *all* lines in the xy-plane given by an equation of the form (13.2) with any intercept a and any slope b. Among them we select the line that approximates the data cloud best in the sense of "least squares". This means the following. For a given line of the form (13.2) we calculate, for every i, the difference between y_i and the value $a + bx_i$. The latter value is the ordinate of the point situated on the line (13.2) with abscissa x_i. We form the sum of the squares of these differences:

$$\left(y_1 - \left(a + bx_1\right)\right)^2 + \left(y_2 - \left(a + bx_2\right)\right)^2 + \ldots + \left(y_n + bx_n\right)^2$$

and look for the values of a and b for which this sum attains its minimum. It is easy to prove that this is the case for the line with intercept $\hat{a}$ and slope $\hat{b}$ given by

$$\hat{b} = s_{xy} / s_x^2 = \rho_{xy} s_y / s_x, \quad \hat{a} = \bar{x} - \hat{b}\bar{y}$$

This line is called the "regression line" for Y on X. As a consequence, the slope of the regression line is positive if and only if the correlation coefficient ρ_{xy} is positive; for uncorrelated variables, the regression line is parallel to the x-axis. In our example with the indicators calculated above, namely $\bar{x} = 53.4074$, $\bar{y} = 74$, $s_x = 23.82$, $s_y = 20.50$, and $\rho_{xy} = 0.2512$, we get

$$\hat{a} = 37.41, \quad \hat{b} = 0.2162$$

The reader should now do the following: First draw the line through the data cloud that seems to approximate the cloud best according to his or her intuition and visual impression; then draw the regression line as calculated; finally compare the two.

A correlation coefficient represents a type of dependence between two variables in a symmetric fashion. A regression line describes how a "dependent" variable depends on an "independent" variable.

Let us finish this section with some remarks about the visual form of descriptive statistics such as histograms and data clouds. They require much thought. They need to be adapted to what they are meant to represent. For example, a so-called "pie chart" may be preferable to a histogram if the focus is on the proportions, or percentages, of the various values within all data. The visual display to be selected must also be as simple as possible. Often an ordinary histogram turns out to be the most instructive. One should avoid unnecessary decorative elements; even colours do very often not contribute to clarity. Three-dimensional representations in perspective of matters that are basically two-dimensional have become fashionable because they are easy to produce by a computer, but they usually impair legibility instead of improving it. Finally, a succinct "legend" as part of a figure is indispensable, indicating for example the meaning of the units on the x- and y-axis. In summary:

A visual display of statistical facts needs to be as simple and clear as possible but it must comprise all elements such as a legend that are necessary so it can be understood by itself.

13.4   Two-by-Two Tables

The second part of Sect. 13.2 and the entire Sect. 13.3 concerned only ordinal variables. Categorical variables demand different tools. We shall restrict ourselves to binary variables. We want to investigate relations between two of them and we use the following example. One of the two variables is the variable "sex" Z defined in Sect. 13.1. The other variable, to be called "high blood pressure" and denoted by W, is derived from the variable Y defined there by distinguishing only diastolic pressure below and above 80 mmHg, more precisely:

$$w_i = 0 \text{ if } y_i \leq 80 \text{ and } w_i = 1 \text{ if } y_i > 80$$

We now write down again the sequence of values of Z and underneath the values of W, which we have derived from those of Y:

$$Z : 0\,0\,0\,1\,0\,1\,1\,1\,1\,0\,1\,1\,1\,1\,0\,1\,0\,0\,1\,1\,0\,1\,0\,1\,1\,0\,0,$$

$$W : 0\,0\,0\,0\,1\,1\,1\,0\,1\,0\,0\,0\,1\,1\,1\,1\,0\,0\,0\,0\,0\,1\,0\,0\,0\,1\,1.$$

Thus, for every patient we have recorded *together*, one over the other, the sex and the hypertension status. By a simple counting exercise we obtain the following four numbers where we have used the abbreviation # for "(cardinal-) number of":

$a = \#$ male patients without hypertension (code 00) = 8,
$b = \#$ male patients with hypertension (code 01) = 4,
$c = \#$ female patients without hypertension (code 10) = 8,
$d = \#$ female patients with hypertension (code 11) = 7.

We display this in the form of a so-called "two-by-two table" see Table 13.1 below, which is a particular "contingency table". Here, $n = a + b + c + d$.

Table 13.1 Gender and hypertension

	$W = 0$	$W = 1$	
$Z = 0$	a	b	$a + b$
$Z = 1$	c	d	$c + d$
	$a + c$	$b + d$	n

We use this table to analyze the relation between Z and W from two different points of view. First we note that the proportion of high blood pressure among males was, after rounding, equal to $b/(a + b) = 4/12 = 0.3333$ but among females it was $c/(c + d) = 7/15 = 0.4667$. Next we find, among those suffering from high blood pressure, a proportion of $b/(b + d) = 4/11 = 0.3636$ male patients whereas among those not afflicted by high blood pressure we have a proportion of $a/(a + c) = 8/16 = 0.5$ males. Both types of analysis point into the same direction, namely that among the 27 patients, females are more prone to high blood pressure.

Let us now focus on a hypothetical situation where the proportion of high blood pressure among males and among females is the same, which means $b/(a + b) = c/(c + d)$. It is easy to prove that this is equivalent to any of the following three statements:

$$b/(b+d) = a/(a+c); \; ad = bc; \; ad/bc = 1$$

Hence the idea of looking at the quantity

$$q = \frac{ad}{bc}$$

in general situations. It is an indicator, which describes a kind of deviation from our hypothetical situation. Again it is easy to see that we have $q > 1$ if and only if the proportion of high blood pressure among males is smaller and $q < 1$ if and only if it is larger than among females. The number q is called the "odds ratio" of the two-by-two table above. Its value in our particular example is 1.75. We shall study it further in Sect. 15.2.

The two different ways of interpreting the data presented above provide a first glimpse at basic techniques of modern epidemiologic studies. Let us again regard the sex Z as the factor and the hypertension status W as the outcome variable. We call the appearance of hypertension in a particular patient a "case" and regard a patient without hypertension as a "control". Then the first way of analyzing the data is close to the idea of a "cohort study" where we have the two cohorts "male" and "female", which are determined by the factor. In both cohorts we measure the proportion of cases and then compare the two with each other. The second way is a kind of rudimentary "case-control study" in which we have two groups defined by the outcome variable, namely "cases" and "controls". In both of them we calculate the proportion of the exposition by the factor ($Z = 1$) and compare the two.

Two-by-two tables play an important role in clinical epidemiology, especially in the evaluation of diagnostic tests, both in daily clinical practice and in screening programmes; see Sect. 19.2.

13.5   The Idea of Inferential Statistics

In this lesson we have derived indicators such as medians, means, standard deviations, correlation coefficients and odds ratios in order to describe essential features of the structure of the given data set. We have hardly drawn any conclusions going beyond the data set itself. In the preceding Lesson 12 the focus was different. From the data in a sample drawn from a larger target population we wanted to infer something about indicators in this target population itself. In particular we have estimated population means by sample means. Thus we were engaged in what is called "inferential statistics".

In the example that has served us throughout the present lesson our target population consisted of 27 consultations in the district hospital of Quynh Phu. This target population is small and not very interesting in itself. A larger and more significant one would consist, for example, of *all* consultations for cardio-vascular diseases in that hospital during the whole year 2010. Important questions would look like this: what was the mean diastolic blood pressure or the influence of the factor "age" on diastolic blood pressure in the entirety of these consultations? To answer such questions we should regard the 27 consultations no longer as the target population but as a sample drawn from a larger target population. However, we need to realize that this sample had not been obtained by an appropriate sampling plan of the type presented in the preceding lesson.

The situation becomes even more complicated when we try to estimate the mean diastolic blood pressure in the entire district of Quynh Phu instead of just one hospital. The sample of 27 consultations is certainly not in any way characteristic of the latter target population because it concerns only consultations and leaves aside healthy people who did not consult in the district hospital; even worse, it comprises only consultations for cardio-vascular diseases! Thus it is subject to the so-called "hospital bias" to be treated in Sects. 20.1 and 27.2.

These discussions show that, in all epidemiologic investigations, we have to keep in mind the following basic statistical principle:

Do not only look at data; also look at the way they were obtained.

In practice, this is often forgotten and replaced by thoughtless use of statistical software.

At the core of the Lessons 14–20 we shall encounter many problems of inferential statistics.

The data sets in epidemiologic investigations are in general relatively small because they concern mainly people and measurements on people; by "relatively small" we may vaguely have in mind "not more than a few thousands". Recently the existence of powerful computers motivated the development of statistical analyses of very large data sets. There have been a few applications in epidemiology, too, but we shall not pursue this.

13.6   Practical Work

1. Draw a "baton" histogram for a sequence of about 50 data of a discrete ordinal variable that you have obtained from medical registers. It is up to you to decide what kind of variable would be appropriate for this exercise. Select the scales on the two axes well and indicate within the figure clearly what they represent: meaning of the values of the variable on the abscissa and of the frequencies (or percentages, proportions,...) on the ordinate. Do the same thing for a categorical variable.
2. Draw the histogram of the variables "age" and "diastolic blood pressure" for the groups and frequencies given in Sect. 13.2.
3. Draw the data cloud as indicated in Sect. 13.3.
4. Familiarize yourself with simple statistical software that may be available to you by calculating the various indicators defined in this lesson with real data obtained from registers or surveys. Note that most programmable pocket calculators contain the necessary software, but you should also use others.

Lesson 14
The Normal Law and Applications: Sample Size, Confidence Intervals, Tests

This lesson presents the fundamental ideas of inferential statistics. It deals with data that stem from either of two sources: – repeated observations that are essentially being done independently of each other under the same conditions; – a sample survey. It is confined to techniques based on the normal law; this permits the use of simple numerical methods.

14.1 The Normal Law

Many histograms evoke the shape of a bell. The histogram of the variable "diastolic blood pressure" in Practical Work no. 2 of Sect. 13.6 is a good example. There is a theorem in the theory of probabilities that explains this observation; it is called the "central limit theorem". As said before, we do not assume knowledge of probability theory in this book, so we describe only the intuitive meaning of the theorem. It says that under certain technical assumptions a random variable which can be thought of as the sum of a large number of components acting more or less independently of each other, will follow approximately a "normal law", to be defined presently. An early application of the normal law around 1800 was to describe the distribution of errors in repeated independent measurements of the same quantity in astronomy and geodesy.

There is a normal law, also called a normal distribution, for every number μ and every positive number σ. It is denoted by $N(\mu,\sigma^2)$ and is given by its so-called "density", which is the function

$$f(x) = \frac{1}{\sigma\sqrt{2\pi}} \exp\left(-\frac{(x-\mu)^2}{2\sigma^2}\right)$$

where "exp" stands for the exponential function. If we draw the curve $y = f(x)$ in the xy-plane, we see that it has indeed the form of a European bell (not an Asian one!),

© Springer Nature Switzerland AG 2019
K. Krickeberg et al., *Epidemiology*, Statistics for Biology and Health,
https://doi.org/10.1007/978-3-030-16368-6_14

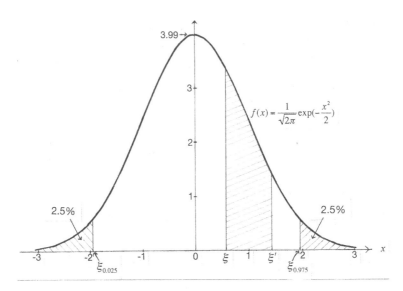

Fig. 14.1 Density of the standard normal distribution. For better visual clarity the numbers 1, 2, 3 and 3.99 in this drawing have been employed to denote the points 0.1, 0.2, 0.3 and 0.399 on the y-axis

albeit with infinite rims; see Fig. 14.1 for the case $\mu = 0$, $\sigma = 1$, with different scales on the x- and the y-axis, which gives the so-called standard normal law. It is symmetric around the point $x = \mu$ where it also takes its maximum. The number μ is the "mean", or "expectation", of $N(\mu, \sigma^2)$ in the sense of probability theory but a rigorous definition of this concept is not needed here.

The area of the surface between the curve f and the x-axis is equal to 1. When x moves away from μ the quantity $f(x)$ decreases rapidly and in fact the faster the smaller σ is. For small values of σ most of the area under the curve is concentrated in the near neighbourhood of μ whereas for large σ it is more "spread out" to the left and the right. Thus σ can be regarded as a measure of the spread of this area. In the sense of probability theory σ is the standard deviation and σ^2 the variance of the normal distribution $N(\mu, \sigma^2)$.

For any two numbers ξ and ξ' such that $\xi < \xi'$ the area under the curve between them is interpreted as the probability of a value between ξ and ξ' with respect to this law; in the case $\mu = 0$, $\sigma = 1$ this is the corresponding shaded area in Fig. 14.1.

An important advantage of the family of laws $N(\mu, \sigma^2)$ is that when we want to obtain such probabilities numerically we can easily reduce the case of a general μ and σ to the case of the standard normal law $N(0,1)$. To this end we standardize a law analogously to the standardization of a variable described further below. There are tables and computer programmes that furnish probabilities for the law $N(0,1)$.

In analogy to the concept of percentiles of a variable defined in Sect. 13.2 we are going to define percentiles of the standard normal law. For any number α between 0 and 1 we denote by ξ_α the number such that the area under the curve to the left of ξ_α

is equal to $\alpha = (\alpha \cdot 100)\%$. Thus we interpret α as the probability of a value less than ξ_α. In most applications we are interested in *small* probabilities α at the "tail" of the distribution, far from the central values around 0. In Fig. 14.1 we have chosen $\alpha = 0.025 = 2.5\%$. In a table of N(0,1) or by a computer programme we find that $\xi_{0.025} = -1.9600$. Since the curve of N(0,1) is symmetric around 0, the probability of a value *greater* than 1.9600 will also be equal to $\alpha = 0.025$. This is 1 minus the probability of a value *less* than 1.9600, which we can express in the form $1.9600 = \xi_{1-\alpha} = \xi_{0.975}$. Finally, the probability of a value less than -1.9600 or greater than 1.9600, in other words of an *absolute* value greater than 1.9600, is equal to $0.05 = 5\%$.

"Normal approximation" of a variable X means, vaguely speaking, that an appropriately chosen histogram of X is close to the density curve of the normal law $N(\mu,\sigma^2)$ for some μ and σ. Usually we can then work with $\mu = \overline{x}$ and $\sigma = s_x$ where $\overline{x}$ and s_x are the mean and the standard deviation of X, that is, we approximate the histogram of X by the density of the law $N(\overline{x}, s_x^2)$.

We can "standardize" the variable X in the following way. If $x_1, x_2, \ldots, x_n$ are the data of X, the standardized variable X^0 is defined as the variable with data $(x_i - \overline{x})/s_x$, $i = 1, \ldots, n$. It shall then admit an approximation by the standard normal law N(0,1) with mean 0 and variance 1. This allows us to use indicators of N(0,1) as approximations to the corresponding indicators of the standardized variable X^0 and derive from them approximations to the indicators of X itself.

The normal approximation becomes useful for data sets of medium or large size. Important applications of the normal approximation will be presented in the next three sections. The general principle looks like this:

Indicators of a normal law are easily available from tables or computer programmes. The corresponding indicators can then be obtained approximately for variables that admit a normal approximation.

Under certain technical assumptions a normal approximation applies in particular to means of data which arise either from observations that are being repeated independently of each other under the same conditions, for example by extraction from a register, or in a sample survey.

The basic ideas of inferential statistics are general and not tied to particular distributions. However, most of the frequently used traditional elementary procedures depend on a normal approximation and this is why we present them in the present lesson.

14.2   Sample Sizes Again

Sample size determination is a vast area because the size of a sample needed in a survey depends on many things: the type and number of indicators to be estimated; the sampling plan to be used; the way we make precise the idea that the estimations should be "good". It would be futile to present technicalities for many different situations.

The basic idea, however, is always the same, and hence we shall restrict ourselves to the frequent case presented at the end of Sect. 12.5, namely the estimation of an unknown small proportion p when we have already some information in the form of an a priori value $\check{p}$.

The formula (12.8) of Sect. 12.5 gives us a first solution of the problem. Regarding the meaning of ε, recall once more that the sample proportion p_S is an estimate of p that we compute *after* having selected the sample S and obtained the data. However, at the stage of planning the survey the sample S is still unknown and depends on chance. Thus p_S, too, depends on chance, and ε denotes its relative standard deviation as discussed in Sects. 12.1 and 12.5. It was this number ε which we had used to express the quality of the estimation procedure.

Often, when planning a survey, we want to describe its quality in a slightly different fashion. Instead of a relative standard deviation, we give ourselves a relative "precision" of the estimate. As we have seen in the examples of Sect. 12.1, an estimate may be very imprecise if we are unlucky enough to obtain by our sampling plan a "bad" sample, but at least we should like this to happen only with a small probability. Thus we fix beforehand the following two numbers according to what we want to achieve by the survey:

- A positive number η to be called the "relative precision". We regard an estimate p_S sufficiently "precise" if $|p_S - p| / p < \eta$.
- A number α such that $0 < \alpha < 1$, to be called the "error probability". We want to find a sample size n such that the probability of an "imprecise" estimate becomes close to α.

We are going to solve this problem for a simple sampling plan. Here the estimate p_S follows indeed approximately a normal law. We shall discuss below some other situations in which this method can also be used.

First, as described in the preceding section, we determine the number ξ such that, for the standard normal law $N(0,1)$, the probability of an absolute value greater than ξ becomes equal to α; in the previous notation, $\xi = \xi_{1-\alpha/2}$. Next, we "standardize" the variable "sample proportion" p_S by subtracting its mean value, which can be shown to be equal to p, and by dividing by its standard deviation, which is close to $\sqrt{p(1-p)/n}$ as follows from the discussion in Sect. 12.5. Since this standardized variable follows approximately the normal law $N(0,1)$ we find, by the definition of ξ, that the probability for the inequality

$$\frac{|p_S - p|}{\sqrt{p(1-p)}} \sqrt{n} > \xi$$

is close to α. This inequality, in turn, is equivalent to

$$\frac{|p_S - p|}{p} > \frac{\xi}{\sqrt{n}} \sqrt{\frac{1-p}{p}}$$

Thus, by the definition of the relative precision η and the error probability α, the expression on the right is identical with η:

$$\frac{\xi}{\sqrt{n}}\sqrt{\frac{1-p}{p}} = \eta$$

Solving for n, neglecting again the proportion p in the difference $1 - p$ and replacing the unknown p by the "a priori" value $\dot{p}$ we finally obtain our result:

The sample size to be used when planning the survey is

$$n \approx \frac{\xi^2}{\eta^2 \dot{p}} \tag{14.1}$$

We may interpret this analogously to the interpretation of the result (12.8) in Sect. 12.5. It implies that a large sample size n is required in the following cases:

- The error probability α is small, that is, the investigator would like to be fairly sure to obtain the precision that he has given himself. In fact, from Fig. 14.1 and the definition of ξ it is obvious that ξ becomes large when α gets small.
- The intended precision measure η is small, which amounts to a very precise estimate.
- The proportion p to be estimated is small.

Let us take up again the example of Sect. 12.5 where $\dot{p} = 0.01 = 1\%$. We strive for a relative precision of $\eta = 0.1 = 10\%$ and again an error probability $\alpha = 0.05 = 5\%$. Then $\xi = 1.96$, hence (14.1) furnishes the sample size $n \approx 38,416$. This large sample size is of course mainly due to the fact that the unknown proportion to be estimated is very small.

The investigator can use (14.1) for balancing out the precision against the error probability and for reducing the sample size if it appears too large to him. For example he may still insist on a fairly small error probability such as 5% but decide that very precise knowledge of p is not so important and that a relative precision of $\eta = 20\%$ instead of 10% would be sufficient. This would divide the needed sample size by the factor 4. On the other hand, if he wants to be even more confident in his estimate and replaces the old error probability $\alpha = 5\%$ by $\alpha = 2\%$, he will find in his table of the normal law or the corresponding computer programme the new value $\xi = 2.3263$ instead of 1.9600, which will increase the required sample size by the factor $(2.3263/1.96)^2 = 1.4087$.

For other sampling plans but a simple one, for example a systematic plan or a two-stage plan where Madow's plan is used at the first stage, a normal approximation and the conclusions we have drawn may not be justified. We have already seen in the first example in Sect. 12.1 that the law of the estimate p_S depends very much on the unknown data in the target population. In practice one still uses the formula

(14.1) for obtaining some information on the order of magnitude of the sample size to be used. However, some thoughts on how to justify a normal approximation in a concrete case are never superfluous.

Finally, if we plan a survey in order to estimate several means or proportions at the same time, the probability of committing an error in at least one of these estimates is of course higher than the error probability for each estimate taken separately. This is often forgotten in practice; we will not enter into the technical details here.

14.3   Estimation and Confidence Intervals

Let us start by going back to some of the discussions in Lesson 13. In its first section, we have described various aspects of a series of data $x_1,\ldots,x_n$ irrespective of their origin. Then, in Sect. 13.5, we have defined the concept of statistical inference where one wants to draw conclusions about a target population based on data that concern only a study population. Let us stress once more, because it is often forgotten in reports on studies and even in research papers, that in any epidemiologic investigation, the target population needs to be specified precisely.

Having obtained the data $x_1,\ldots,x_n$ the investigator starts analyzing and evaluating them. He will, for example, calculate among others the mean $\bar{x}$ and the variance s^2 of the data as defined at the end of Sect. 13.1. Attention: if the data have arisen from a sample survey, there is an unavoidable confusion of notations because $\bar{x}$ now stands for the *sample* mean and not, as in Lesson 12, for the *population* mean; likewise, s is now the standard deviation in the sample, not in the population. The two quantities $\bar{x}$ and s in the present sense are those with which the investigator is actually working whereas the population mean and population standard deviation are unknown quantities about which he would like to find out something.

It is important to realize that in the underlying theory, we regard the data as the result of a random process. When they stem from a sample survey, this is implicit in the definition of a sampling plan. When we extract them from registers, the way we do it also usually involves chance. Moreover there are always some random elements in the data themselves by their very nature. For example, the way a disease has evolved, the reasons for which the patient decides to consult the health facility and the measurement of his various symptoms depend on chance. In practice, when the investigator uses certain procedures, often in the form of statistical software, in order to analyze his data, he treats them as fixed numbers. However, understanding their random origin is indispensable for knowing *why* these procedures are applied and *how* the results are to be interpreted. For simplicity, we shall use the same notations for the given data and indicators on the one hand and for the corresponding random variables on the other hand, but it will always be clear from the context whether we consider the data as fixed numbers or as numbers depending on chance.

The first concepts we intend to study are "estimation" and "confidence intervals". We would like to estimate an unknown mean μ, which we usually imagine to be the population mean of a variable in the target population. For example, μ may be the average number of cigarettes smoked by the entire adult population of Vietnam in the year 2017. What we know are the numbers of cigarettes smoked by n people selected somehow, that is the data $x_1,\ldots,x_n$. We use the mean $\bar{x}$ of these data to estimate μ.

In Sect. 12.1 in the realm of sample surveys, we have described the "quality" of an estimation procedure with the help of its mean square error M^2. We do the same for data collected in other ways, for example for data obtained independently of each other under the same conditions, using the same definition of M^2. Again, we call M the "standard deviation" of the estimation of μ by the estimator $\bar{x}$, and M/μ the "relative standard deviation". They indicate how good our method of estimating is.

We recall from Sect. 12.5 that for data obtained by a simple sampling plan, the quantity s/n is a "reasonable" estimate of M. A similar statement is often true for data that arise in other ways as sketched before.

Let us look at the example of diastolic blood pressure of all patients consulting the outpatient ward of the district hospital of Quynh Phu in spring 2010 for some cardio-vascular problem. For the data set Y in Sect. 13.1 we had $n = 27$, $\bar{y} = 74$ and, from the end of Sect. 13.2, $s = s_y = 20.50$. This furnishes the estimate $s_y / \sqrt{n} = 20.5 / \sqrt{27} = 3.95$ of M. Therefore the *estimated* relative standard deviation of the estimation procedure is equal to $3.95/74 \approx 5.3\%$. Thus we may say that for most practical purposes our estimation procedure for μ is quite good. This is mainly due to the fact that we have a fairly large number of data, namely 27, at our disposal.

We shall now, in analogy to the preceding Section, adopt a different point of view and treat the problem in terms of the concepts of "precision" and "error probability".

To this end, we construct an interval around the estimate $\bar{x}$ with a lower bound $\bar{x} - \vartheta\left(s / \sqrt{n}\right)$ and an upper bound $\bar{x} + \vartheta\left(s / \sqrt{n}\right)$, written as usual in the form

$$\left[\bar{x} - \vartheta\left(s / \sqrt{n}\right),\ \bar{x} + \vartheta\left(s / \sqrt{n}\right)\right]. \tag{14.2}$$

Here ϑ is a positive number still to be determined, which will represent the "precision" of the estimate. This interval depends on the data through $\bar{x}$ and s. It can be calculated if ϑ has been fixed and the data are known. In the underlying theory, though, it is a "random interval" because $\bar{x}$ and s depend on chance. We are interested in the probability that the "true" mean μ is situated inside it, which amounts to saying that the difference between $\bar{x}$ and μ is, in absolute value, not larger than $\vartheta\left(s / \sqrt{n}\right)$. We should of course like this probability to be high, that is, close to one, and in practice we therefore pose the problem the other way round. For a given small probability α which we shall call the "error probability" or the "risk", for example $\alpha = 5\%$, we want to determine the number ϑ in such a way that the random interval (14.2) covers the unknown fixed mean μ with the probability $1 - \alpha$. We then call (14.2) a "confidence interval" for μ on the "level" $1 - \alpha$ and the boundaries of this interval are called the "confidence bounds" for μ on this level.

In order to solve the problem of finding ϑ for a given error probability α we shall use the so-called t-distribution with $n - 1$ degrees of freedom. We will not give its definition here because in practice one uses tables or software for this distribution in much the same way as for the normal distribution. Suffice it to say that the t-distribution with $n - 1$ degrees of freedom is derived from the standard normal distribution. It is symmetric around 0 and for large n it is sufficiently close to the standard normal distribution to be replaced by it; in normal practice it is being done as soon as $n \geq 20$.

The intuitive idea which motivated the use of a t-distribution is simple. Suppose the data $x_1, \ldots, x_n$ are the result of n observations that all follow the same normal law and are independent of each other. We want to "standardize" $\bar{x}$ as described in Sect. 14.1 by dividing it by its standard deviation but since this is not known we replace it by its estimate based on the same data, namely by $s / \sqrt{n}$. Then it can be shown that the quantity

$$\frac{\bar{x} - \mu}{s} \sqrt{n} \tag{14.3}$$

regarded as a random variable follows the t-distribution with $n - 1$ degrees of freedom.

We now proceed analogously to what we did in the preceding section. In a table of this distribution we look up the value ϑ such that the random variable (14.3) is larger than ϑ with the probability $\alpha/2$, which is equivalent to saying that (14.3) in absolute value is larger than ϑ with the probability α. In many practical situations we can work from the beginning with the standard normal distribution instead of a t-distribution.

Let us construct the confidence interval on the level 95% derived from the 27 data Y of Sect. 13.1. We had found $\bar{y} = 74$ and $s = s_y = 20.50$. The table of the t-distribution with 26 degrees of freedom gives us $\vartheta = 2.056$ whereas the one of N(0,1) furnishes, as we already know, $\vartheta = 1.960$. We shall simply work with $\vartheta = 2$. In fact, using $\vartheta = 1.960$ as one often finds it done in reports and research papers is ridiculous because it gives the illusion of a high precision whereas the whole process contains many approximations and sources of errors. With $\vartheta = 2$ we obtain the confidence interval, rounded again to the nearest integers, from 66 to 82. It is then customary to say that, on the confidence level 95%, the true mean μ is situated between 66 and 82. The usual statistical software provides confidence intervals directly from the data and the risk α.

As in the problem of choosing a sample size, the investigator needs to weigh precision against a high level of confidence. For example, if he wants to be very sure of his result as expressed by the confidence interval, he may opt for a confidence level of 99% instead of 95%, that is, an error probability of only 1% instead of 5%. By using again a table of the t-distribution with 26 degrees of freedom he finds $\vartheta = 2.779$ while the standard normal distribution would give him $\vartheta = 2.576$. To be on the safe side, he uses the larger, and rounded, value $\vartheta = 2.8$, which furnishes, after rounding to the nearest integer, the confidence interval [63, 85] to be compared with the confidence interval [66, 82] on the confidence level 95%. The latter is narrower and gives more precise bounds but with less certainty.

To resume the basic ideas in a somewhat vague fashion:

An estimate of an unknown parameter is a number calculated from the data, which one expects to be in general close to the "true value" of the parameter. The quality of an estimation procedure is usually described by its mean square error.

A confidence interval for an unknown parameter is an interval calculated from the data that covers the true value with a certain probability, which is called its confidence level. The length of the confidence interval is a measure of the precision of the information contained in the statement: "The parameter is situated in the confidence interval"; a small interval means high precision.

Looking finally again at the particular case of a binary variable we recall that $\bar{x} = p_S$ is the proportion of the values 1 among the observed data and that $s \approx \sqrt{p_S(1 - p_S)}$; these values are to be used when calculating the confidence interval (14.2).

14.4   Tests of Statistical Hypotheses

Confidence intervals provide fairly complete information on an unknown "parameter" μ and should in general be the preferred form of stating the result of an elementary evaluation of data. Sometimes, however, we are only interested in a partial aspect, to be expressed as a "hypothesis". For example suppose that we should like to know whether, as a result of a health education programme, the average diastolic blood pressure μ among patients consulting the outpatient ward of the district hospital of Quynh Phu for cardio-vascular diseases has fallen below 80 mmHg. This is our hypothesis to be tested, written as

$$H_1 : \mu < 80 \, (\text{mmHg})$$

for historical reasons it is also being called the "alternative hypothesis".

We then use a "statistical test".

A statistical test is a rule that tells us when to accept or not to accept H_1, depending on the data.

We also consider the "null hypothesis"

$$H_0 : \mu \geq 80 \, (\text{mmHg})$$

It may of course happen that, by a test, we accept H_1 although it is wrong, that is, when H_0 is true. We should like to find a test such that, if H_1 is wrong, we accept it only with a small probability given in advance.

To make this idea precise we fix again a small "error probability" α and look up, in a table of the t-distribution with $n - 1$ degrees of freedom, the number ϑ such that a variable which follows this distribution takes a value greater than ϑ with the probability α (not $\alpha/2$ as in the preceding section!). In other words, ϑ is the $(1 - \alpha)100$-percentile of this distribution. If n is sufficiently large, we use a table of the standard normal distribution instead. Then we apply the following test:

$$\Theta : \text{Accept } H_1 \text{ if and only if } \overline{x} + \vartheta \frac{s}{\sqrt{n}} < 80.$$

It can be shown that if H_0 is true, that is, if $\mu \geq 80$, the probability of accepting H_1 by the test Θ is indeed less than or equal to α; in the particular case $\mu = 80$ it is equal to α. More generally:

A number α is called an error probability or "risk" of a test Θ if, in case H_0 is true, the probability of accepting H_1 by Θ is less than or equal to α; sometimes, one also says that Θ is a test on the "level" $1 - \alpha$.

The test Θ above is called the "t-test" or "Student's test". Student was a pseudonym of the British statistician W. S. Gosset who published his basic result in 1908. Let us try to understand the reasoning behind his test first from the point of view of estimation and then from that of confidence bounds. The population mean $\overline{x}$ is a reasonable estimate of μ. Hence if $\overline{x}$ turns out to be distinctly smaller than 80, we will be inclined to deduce that μ, too, is smaller than 80 which would mean that H_1 would be true. The question arises: *how much* smaller than 80 does $\overline{x}$ have to be in order to allow us to conclude, with a given error probability, that $\mu < 80$? Student's test Θ gives the answer. We had already alluded to this type of questions in Sect. 3.1.

The reasoning behind the test also becomes clear if we go back to the construction of confidence intervals. The quantity $\overline{x} + \vartheta s / \sqrt{n}$ is the upper bound of the confidence interval for μ with the risk 2α; we had in fact constructed this confidence interval in such a way that $\mu \leq \overline{x} + \vartheta s / \sqrt{n}$ holds with the probability $1 - \alpha$. Now, this inequality together with the inequality above in the definition of the test Θ which leads us to accept H_1, implies $\mu < 80$, and this means indeed that H_1 is true.

In practice, one often chooses the error probability $\alpha = 0.05 = 5\%$, following Sir R. A. Fisher, one of the founding fathers of modern inferential statistics. Other error probabilities are also being used, for example $\alpha = 0.01$ if one wants to be very sure of a correct conclusion when the test leads to accepting H_1.

It is important to realize that if we do not accept the hypothesis H_1 by our test Θ, we cannot simply affirm that it is wrong, in other words, that the null hypothesis H_0 is true. Not accepting H_1 only means that we remain ignorant about its validity because the data have not conveyed sufficient information. As in most scientific investigations we want to "discover" an effect, for example the decrease of the average diastolic blood pressure below 80 mmHg as a result of health education, if it really exists. Therefore one defines the "power" of a test as the probability of

Table 14.1 Student's test on various levels

$\alpha \cdot 100\%$	ϑ	$y + \vartheta s_y / \sqrt{n}$	Accept H_1?
1%	2.479	83.78	No
2.5%	2.056	82.11	No
5%	1.706	80.73	No
10%	1.315	79.19	Yes

accepting H_1 if it is true. This probability still depends, in our example, on the unknown value μ.

Sometimes one speaks about a "positive" result of the test if one can accept the hypothesis. "Negative" then only means that one has not been able to accept the hypothesis but the effect in question may nevertheless exist. In that case, the negative result is due to a low power of the test, especially when the samples are small.

High power is a desirable feature of a test. We can imagine many other tests besides the t-test for testing, with a small error probability, the hypothesis H_1 against the null hypothesis H_0. For example the test "Never accept H_1 whatever the data are" has the error probability 0 but it is obviously of no use; it has power 0. It can be proved that under certain conditions the t-test has, whatever the value $\mu < 80$ may be, the highest power among all tests with an error probability below a given number.

Let us now try out Student's test with several risks α and the data Y of Sect. 13.1; recall once more that $\bar{y} = 74$ and $s = s_y = 20.50$. The results are presented in Table 14.1, based on the t-distribution with $n - 1 = 26$ degrees of freedom.

It is good statistical practice to determine a test and in particular its error probability α *before* evaluating and if possible even *before* collecting the data; this should be part of planning the study. Nevertheless one often computes *afterwards* from the data the smallest risk with which one can accept the hypothesis H_1 by a t-test; this is called the "p-value" of the data for H_1. In our example we see from Table 14.1 that the p-value is situated between 5 and 10%. To find its precise value, we solve the equation $\bar{y} + \vartheta s_y / \sqrt{n} = 80$ for ϑ, which yields $\vartheta = 1.521$, and then obtain from a table of the t-distribution with 26 degrees of freedom the probability of surpassing ϑ, namely $0.073 = 7.3\%$; this is the p-value of our study.

Let us summarize the essence of the concept of testing in a slightly less precise way:

A statistical test Θ of a given hypothesis H_1 is a rule that tells us when to accept or not to accept H_1, depending on the data. Its error probability, or risk, is the probability of accepting H_1 when H_1 is wrong while its power is the probability of accepting H_1 when it is true. These numbers do not depend on the data but only on the test.

By contrast, the p-value is computed from the data. It concerns tests of a given form and is the smallest risk of all these tests which allow to accept the hypothesis H_1.

Hence a small p-value means that we can accept H_1 by a test of small error probability and thus regard the result as "significant". Again, a p-value less than or equal to 5% is usually considered "small" in this sense.

Inferential statistics is a vast domain with many techniques adapted to such and such problem. Relatively new areas such as inference from very large data sets appear. The basic ideas that we have presented still permeate most of the problems encountered in epidemiologic practice. The reader should not try to memorize techniques for handling all possible variants of the situation that we have described. Instead, faced with a particular investigation to be planned, he or she should try to *understand* the essential aspects, look for the specific techniques needed in the particular case at hand, and, as soon as things seem to become a bit complicated, consult a statistician *before* writing the plan for his or her study.

Regarding in particular statistical tests we have noted in the beginning of the present section that other inferential methods are in general preferable. In fact the field of testing statistical hypotheses is dying, both as a field of research and as an arsenal of tools for practice. The only reason for having sketched it here is that it is still being applied in certain epidemiologic investigations; therefore the readers of this book must understand its principles. The authors of this book hope that in its next edition the present Sect. 14.4 can be discarded completely!

14.5   Practical Work

1. In the year 2006 a survey was conducted in the district Vu Thu of the province of Thaí Bình in order to estimate the proportion p of persons aged over 15 who suffered from depressions. In a sample of 2969 subjects, their proportion was $p_S = 0.044 = 4.4\%$. Construct a confidence interval for p on the level 95%.
2. The purpose of a survey in a given population of children was to find out whether one could assert that its coverage p by the BCG-vaccination (Sect. 5.3) exceeded 80%. A sample of 200 children was drawn by an appropriate sampling plan; 176 children in this sample had the scar that testified to the vaccination. Can you accept the hypothesis H_1: $p > 80\%$ against the null hypothesis H_0: $p \leq 80\%$ with an error probability less than or equal to 0.01? What was the p-value of the data for these hypotheses? Should you use a t- or the standard normal distribution?

Lesson 15
Basic Concepts of Epidemiology

The basic concepts of epidemiology are presented first for a target population and then for a study population.

15.1 Concepts About a Population that are Independent of Any Study

Many concepts of epidemiology such as incidence or prevalence of a disease, mortality and risk factors have already appeared in previous lessons. Their meaning was sufficiently clear to allow a preliminary discussion of the basic principles of epidemiology, of its role in public health and of the main issues in the epidemiology of infectious diseases but a rigorous definition was missing. Without rigorous definitions, however, it is impossible to conduct epidemiologic studies of any value. Hence we are now going to state the main definitions while restricting ourselves to the fundamental ones and not entering into the many ramifications that exist.

An investigator who is planning or evaluating a study is almost always dealing only with part of the target population in which he or she is interested. The data concern only the study population, which is a sample from the target population, and this is what he or she focuses on in practice. Sometimes, both in the study plan and in the final report on the study, the target population is not even mentioned and apparently forgotten. However, the purpose of a study is to get to know something about the whole target population with a view of applying this knowledge. Therefore, in the following we shall rigorously distinguish between concepts that concern a whole population, independently of any study, and concepts tied to a study.

We shall look at a specific human target population and shall denote it by U as we had done in Sect. 12.2; for example U may consist of all inhabitants of the province of Thaí Bình. We focus on a well-defined disease D such as chronic obstructive bronchitis and a moment of time t, for example the 1st March 2016.

The prevalence of D in U at the moment t is the number of diagnosed cases of D that exist in U at that moment.

© Springer Nature Switzerland AG 2019
K. Krickeberg et al., *Epidemiology*, Statistics for Biology and Health,
https://doi.org/10.1007/978-3-030-16368-6_15

This prevalence is sometimes called a "total" prevalence to distinguish it from a "prevalence density", which is a proportion. The prevalence density of D in U at the moment t is the total prevalence divided by the population number N of U at the moment t. Thus it is a number between 0 and 1, but often it is given as a percentage, or number of cases per 1000, or per 10,000, per 100,000 people etc., depending on what is more practical. For a very frequent disease such as seasonal influenza, one might use a percentage whereas for a very rare disease such as Churg-Strauss' disease, indicating the number of existing cases per 100,000 people would be more illuminating.

The prevalence density conveys in general a clearer picture of the importance or burden of the disease than the total prevalence.

Unfortunately, the terminology varies a lot. Some authors mean by "prevalence" what we have called the prevalence density. Others talk about "prevalence rate" instead of prevalence density, which is, however, confusing since "rate" in general refers to a period of time and not to a particular moment. Still others use the term "relative prevalence" to denote a prevalence density. We have indeed employed the epithet "relative" in Lessons 12, 13 and 14 in a similar sense but in epidemiology proper as exposed in the present and the following lessons it has a different meaning in concepts such as "relative risk", which will be defined below. The term "density" in the present context, although less common, is unambiguous and also conveys a certain intuitive impression.

Prevalence means the number of cases that *exist* at a given *moment* whereas incidence, to be defined presently, is the number of *new* cases that *appear* during a given *period*. Thus, let J be a certain period, for example the month of March 2016.

The incidence of D in U during J is defined as the number of new cases of D that are diagnosed in U during J.

The "incidence density" is the incidence divided by the population number. It is also frequently called "incidence rate"; here the use of the expression "rate" is better justified since it refers to a period of time, namely to J. Note that the population number may change during this period. The number of inhabitants of the province of Thaí Bình on the 1st March 2016 is not the same as on the 31st March. It is customary to use the number of inhabitants at the middle of the period J, the so-called "midpoint"; in our example it is the 15th March 2016.

Often the health situation at hand is "stationary", or "stable" in time, that is, circumstances do not change much with time. In such a situation there is a simple relation between incidence, prevalence and average duration of the disease from the moment of the first diagnosis to recovery or death, namely

$$\text{prevalence} \approx \text{incidence} \times \text{average duration.}$$

Here, the unit of time in which the average duration is expressed must be the length of the period for which the incidence is defined, for example a week or a month. It is easy to prove this relation; see Practical Work 1, below.

The definition of "mortality" in the population U during a period J is analogous to that of an incidence, namely the number of deaths in U during J. In practice, one usually chooses for J a calendar year. The corresponding "mortality density", for example the number of deaths per 100,000 inhabitants during the period J, is defined accordingly. It is also called "mortality rate" or "death rate". As before we may say that indicators representing densities are usually more revealing than total ones.

Mortality in this sense means "mortality from all causes". In epidemiology we are also interested in mortalities from specific causes. An example would be the total mortality due to pulmonary tuberculosis in the province of Thai Binh during the year 2016, which is the number of deaths due to this disease that occurred in Thai Binh during that year. Again, we derive case-specific mortality *rates* by dividing the absolute mortalities by the number of inhabitants, for example on the 1st July 2016.

A concept of a different nature is that of the "case-fatality" of a given disease, for example for influenza $A|H_1N_1$:

Case-fatality of a disease D is the proportion of the cases with a fatal issue among all cases of D.

According to WHO, until the 15th June 2009 there had been 35,928 confirmed cases of this type of influenza in the whole world of which 163 cases resulted in death. Hence the corresponding case-fatality was equal to $163/35,928 = 0.004537 = 0.4537\%$. Case-fatality is a characteristic of a specific disease but it obviously also depends on the population and the period of time in which it is being considered. Social and economic conditions as well as factors like the general health of the population and its immune status may influence case-fatalities.

Of course, measuring a case-fatality like that above rests on knowing the underlying incidences and cases of death, which in turn depends on correct diagnoses and reliable reporting. For example, on the 25th October 2009 WHO published the figures of 440,000 cases of $A|H_1N_1$ to have occurred in the world until then and 5700 deaths among them, which gives now a case-fatality of 1.3%. This increase of the case-fatality could be explained by several phenomena that may act together. For example, the real case-fatality may indeed have increased; or more cases of an influenza-like syndrome may have been declared as influenza $A|H_1N_1$ than before, perhaps because of improved diagnostic facilities or political considerations; or more cases of deaths from an influenza-like syndrome are now correctly diagnosed as due to influenza $A|H_1N_1$.

The concepts defined until now represent "static" aspects of an epidemiologic situation in the sense that they do not describe changes in time. We have been looking only at an incidence in a *fixed* period of time or at a prevalence at a *fixed* moment. In order to investigate changes in time we could simply compare incidences in different periods or prevalence at different moments. There are also more sophisticated concepts to deal with changes in time. They centre on the concept of a "rate" mentioned above, but we shall not treat them in the present first introduction.

We shall now get to the heart of the matter, namely to the description of the "influence" of factors on health-related variables; recall the definition of epidemiology stated in Sect. 1.3. It is a vast field but nevertheless all ways of analyzing the influence of a factor are oriented by what we may call the *essence of epidemiology*:

We describe the influence of a factor on an outcome variable by *comparing* with each other indicators about the outcome variable for different levels of the factor.

For example, we compare the mortality by lung cancer among smokers with that among non-smokers.

Most of the essential ideas can be explained in the case of binary variables, and in the present book we shall restrict ourselves to this case. Thus we have in the first place the outcome variable; we call its two values "diseased" and "non-diseased". Here the term "diseased" may for example be interpreted in the sense of a prevalence or of an incidence depending on the problem at hand. Instead of "diseased" we may also have outcomes such as "died" or "feeling worse". We shall illustrate the concepts with the help of the following example where we are dealing with a prevalence: the target population U is the entire adult population of the province of Thai Binh on the 1st January 2016. A diseased person is somebody who suffered on that day from confirmed pulmonary tuberculosis. In this way, the target population U is divided into two parts, or "subpopulations", namely the part D_1 of all diseased people and the part D_0 of all non-diseased people.

D_0 and D_1 are determined by the outcome variable. For the risk factor, we choose the following example: a person is said to be "exposed" if he or she had at most primary education; the person is considered "non-exposed" if he or she has obtained at least secondary education. Thus U is divided into the subpopulation E_1 of all exposed people and the subpopulation E_0 of all non-exposed people; they are determined by the risk factor.

As usual we employ the symbol # to mean "number of". In our example, $N = \#U$ is the number of adult inhabitants of the province of Thai Binh on the 1st January 2016, $\#D_1$ is the total prevalence of pulmonary tuberculosis then and there, and $\#D_1/\#U$ is the corresponding prevalence density. It is sometimes illuminating to think of prevalence densities as "risks", or "probabilities", of diseases. Thus, $\#D_1/\#U$ would be interpreted as the risk, or the probability, of an adult inhabitant of Thai Binh selected at random of suffering on the 1st January 2016 from pulmonary tuberculosis.

We now look separately at the prevalence density of pulmonary tuberculosis among exposed and among non-exposed subjects, and then compare the two. The number of diseased persons among exposed subjects is, in simple mathematical notation, $\#(D_1 \cap E_1)$; recall that $D_1 \cap E_1$ stands for the intersection of D_1 and E_1. This is the set of all persons who belong to both D_1 and E_1, in other words, who were both exposed and diseased. Therefore the prevalence density, or "risk", of the disease among exposed subjects is

$$p = \#\left(D_1 \cap E_1 \right) / \# E_1$$

Analogously, we have the risk of the disease among non-exposed subjects, namely

$$p' = \#\left(D_1 \cap E_0\right) / \# E_0$$

There are several ways of comparing the two risks p and p'. In qualitative terms, if $p > p'$, we would say that the exposure has increased the risk of the disease. Among quantitative measures of the influence of the exposure the "risk ratio"

$$r = p / p'$$

is the most useful and widely used one in public health. For example, if $r = 1.3$, we may state that, for a given number of subjects such as 10,000, there are 30% more cases among 10,000 exposed persons than among 10,000 non-exposed ones.

A risk ratio is also frequently being called a "relative risk".

Sometimes, one uses the "risk difference" $p - p'$ for comparing the two risks. A few authors call it the "attributable risk" but others mean something different by this term; hence it is better not to employ it.

The risk ratio r determines a quantity that plays an important role in preventive health. It is called the "aetiological fraction among the exposed" and is defined as

$$\eta = \frac{p - p'}{p} = 1 - \frac{1}{r}$$

The aetiological fraction among the exposed represents the proportion of cases among exposed subjects that can be considered as being *due* to the exposure.

It is also known as the "*attributable* fraction among the exposed" or "exposed attributable fraction" for short. In our example, we may indeed ask ourselves which proportion of the cases of pulmonary tuberculosis among people without secondary education have really been caused by this factor, and would not have come about anyway even without the exposure. An example of even greater importance for public health is lung cancer and smoking. Which proportion of lung cancer among smokers is *due* to their habit of smoking? There have been many studies to answer this question and all of them give values of η not far from $1 = 100\%$; see Sect. 22.3.

Finding a high aetiological fraction among the exposed can be a powerful motivation to start preventive measures. The concept also plays an important role in preventive health in a different way. The idea is to regard the *absence* of prevention as an exposure. To have something concrete in mind, let us look at a vaccination against a disease such as measles. Dividing the population U into a non-vaccinated and a vaccinated part is not what is actually happening in a normal immunization programme. We shall therefore adopt again the theoretical approach that we have already used in Sect. 5.3 when we defined the "efficacy" of a vaccination procedure. In this approach we first imagine that *no* subject of U was vaccinated and denote by p the risk of the disease in this case. Analogously we denote by p' the risk of the disease if *everybody* in U was vaccinated. Then the aetiological fraction η among the exposed as defined above can be rewritten as

$$\eta = \frac{pN - p'N}{pN}$$

where $N = \#U$ stands again for the number of people in U. Here, pN is the number of cases if nobody gets vaccinated, $p'N$ the number of cases if everybody gets vaccinated, hence $pN - p'N$ is the number of cases *prevented* by the vaccination and therefore η is the proportion of cases of the disease prevented by the vaccination among all subjects that would have fallen ill if there had been no vaccination. This is indeed the efficacy of the vaccination procedure as defined in Sect. 5.3. The reasoning used here is sometimes called "counterfactual" because in reality we cannot vaccinate and at the same time not vaccinate the entire population U; it is a theoretical argument. In Sect. 18.2 we shall look at the practical aspects of estimating η.

Generalizing this idea slightly we may state:

For a preventive measure that applies to individual subjects of the target population, its efficacy is the aetiological fraction among the exposed if one interprets "exposed" as "absence of the preventive measure".

For examples in addition to vaccinations we may think of a preventive drug intake against malaria, or calcium plus vitamin D tablets to prevent osteoporosis.

One also defines the "attributable fraction *in the population*" or "population attributable fraction" but we shall not treat this here.

In addition to the risk difference $p - p'$ and the risk ratio $r = p/p'$ one often uses a third quantity for comparing the two risks p among exposed and p' among non-exposed; it is called the "odds-ratio" and will be denoted by q. We first define the "odds" of any risk p as the ratio $p/(1 - p)$, that is, the risk of being or falling ill relative to the risk of not being or falling ill.

The odds ratio is the quotient of the odds of p and of p', in a formula

$$q = \frac{p}{1-p} : \frac{p'}{1-p'}$$

In order to study the relationship between the odds ratio q and the risk ratio r we rewrite this definition in the form

$$q = r\frac{1-p'}{1-p} \tag{15.1}$$

We look separately at the two cases $p > p'$ and $p < p'$. The first case is the one where the exposition increases the risk. In this case, the formula (15.1) implies that $1 < r < q$. In the second case where the exposition decreases the risk, we deduce from (15.1) that $q < r < 1$. Thus, q is indeed a sensible indicator of an influence of the exposition on prevalence or incidence, respectably. However, it is much less suited than the risk ratio for applications in public health, for example as a basis of an intervention programme. The relation (15.1) also shows that we cannot obtain r from q or conversely; the quantitative relation between the two depends on the risks p and p' themselves. For example if q is much larger than 1, the risk ratio r may still be close to 1.

The odds ratio derives its importance from the fact that in so-called case-control studies, to be treated in Lesson 20, it can be estimated directly, which is not the case for the risk ratio. Moreover it follows from the relation (15.1) above that for *small* risks p and p' the two quantities r and q are close to each other. It is indeed the domain of *rare* diseases where the odds ratio plays its main role.

15.2   Epidemiologic Studies

Simple epidemiologic studies have already appeared in Lessons 3 and 11–14. In the present section we shall remain in the framework of a target population U in which there is, on the one hand, a risk factor that divides U into the set E_1 of "exposed" and the set E_0 of "non-exposed" subjects, and on the other hand an outcome variable by which U is divided into the set D_1 of "diseased" subjects and the set D_0 of "non-diseased" ones.

Suppose now that we have executed a study. It may have been a sample survey, or we may have extracted data from registers, or conducted a more refined study of the type to be treated in Lessons 16–20. Whatever the study may have been, we have always got a *sample* from U, that is, a certain subpopulation S of U which is called the "study population". For every person in S we know whether he or she had been exposed or not and whether he or she is diseased or not. We can record this information in coded form. For the exposure variable, we let the value 1 mean "exposed" and 0 mean "not exposed". The value 1 of the outcome variable will mean "diseased" and the value 0 will mean "not diseased". Then, given a person in S, the code 11 stands for "exposed and diseased", 10 for "exposed and not diseased", 01 for "not exposed and diseased" and 00 for "not exposed and not diseased". These four pairs of numbers, for all persons in S, are the *data* that we have obtained by the study.

We are interested in the size of these four categories, that is, in the number of subjects in them. We represent these sizes in a two-by-two table similar to Table 13.1, namely Table 15.1.

Table 15.1   A two-by-two table

	Diseased: 1	Not diseased: 0	Total
Exposed: 1·	a	b	$a + b$
Not exposed: 0·	c	d	$c + d$
Total	$a + c$	$b + d$	n

Here, for example, a denotes the number of subjects in the study who are both exposed and diseased, coded by 11; analogously b, c and d. Finally, $n = \#S = a + b + c + d$ is the total number of persons in the study.

These numbers now allow us to define and to calculate numbers that concern the study population S and correspond to the indicators defined in the preceding section for the entire target population U. Here is a list of them. We use the same notations as before but with the subscript "s" attached. In his mind the reader should add everywhere "in the study population". Instead of "prevalence", we should of course have to write "incidence" or "mortality" depending on the type of problem.

$a + c$: (Total) prevalence.

$(a + c)/n$: Prevalence density.

$p_s = a/(a + b)$: Prevalence density (risk) among the exposed.

$p_s' = c/(c + d)$: Prevalence density (risk) among the non-exposed.

$p_s - p_s'$: Risk difference.

$$r_s = \frac{p_s'}{p_s} = \frac{a(c+d)}{c(a+b)} : \text{Risk ratio (relative risk).}$$

$$\eta_s = \frac{p_s - p_s'}{p_s} = 1 - (1/r_s) : \text{Aetiological (attributable) fraction among the exposed.}$$

$$q_s = \frac{p_s}{1 - p_s} : \frac{p_s'}{1 - p_s'} = \frac{ad}{bc} : \text{Odds ratio.}$$

It is of utmost importance, however, to realize that these are only formal definitions. They may not have any useful interpretation beyond the sample itself. For example the risk ratio in the study population may tell us nothing about the risk ratio in the target population. Here is again the fundamental principle of epidemiologic studies already stated in Sect. 13.5:

The evaluation and interpretation of the data in an epidemiologic study depends not only on the data themselves, but also on the way they had been obtained, that is, on the form of the study.

In the following lessons we shall see what this means in concrete situations and in detail. Basically there are three ways to obtain data:

In a *cross-sectional* study, subjects are selected independently of their exposure and of their disease status.

In a *cohort* study, one selects, independently of each other, two so-called "cohorts", namely a sample of exposed subject and a sample of non-exposed subjects.

In a *case-control* study, one selects, independently of each other, a sample of "cases", that is, of diseased subjects, and a sample of "controls", that is, of non-diseased subjects. This is done independently of their exposure status.

In order to emphasize the essentials, we have not mentioned the time dimension of a study. In a cross-sectional study, the disease status to be observed usually concerns the past or present, depending on the type of problem at hand. Most cohort studies deal with a disease status in the future; one "follows" the two cohorts during a certain time and observes how their disease status evolves. In a case-control study, the investigator observes the exposure status in the past or present. We shall come back to this in the Lessons 16, 17 and 20.

As said above, most basic concepts of epidemiology can be presented in the simple framework of a single binary exposure variable and a single binary outcome variable. Hence we shall remain in this framework also in the next few lessons. There is, however, one fundamental concept that pervades almost all of epidemiology and that concerns the interplay of at least three variables. It is called "confounding" and will be treated in Lesson 21.

In real studies one often investigates several exposures and several outcomes together but the underlying ideas are still the same. This is in particular true in the examples in the later Lessons 22–26 and we shall not point it out every time again.

15.3   Objectives of Studies, Causative Factors, Aetiology

In the preceding session we have distinguished three types of studies by the way they recruit their study population. There is also a distinction determined by their *objectives*. It corresponds largely to the distinction between various types of epidemiology as defined in the Sects. 1.2, 2.2 and 18.1, for example descriptive epidemiology and analytic epidemiology.

The objectives also determine another kind of distinguishing between two basic types of epidemiologic studies, namely between observational and experimental ones. In an "observational study" we investigate the influence of factors that exist already and are not constructed especially for the study. The factors in our list given in Sect. 1.5 are of this type except those in the last category. An "experimental study" analyzes the result of factors that are created for the study. The most important types of such factors are curative and preventive treatments; they are the subject of *clinical trials* (see Lesson 18).

Among observational studies one distinguishes sometimes between *descriptive* studies on the one hand and *analytic* ones as noted above. This distinction is a bit vague, though. A descriptive study puts less emphasis on the influence of risk factors; sometimes it is a sample survey as defined in Sect. 12.4. An analytic study is meant to examine associations between risk factors and health outcomes, in particular for possible causal relations.

Thus let us now look again at the aetiology of diseases and the role epidemiology plays in it. We have already stressed in Sect. 1.6 that epidemiologic indicators and the results of epidemiologic studies are of a statistical nature and do not imply that such and such determinant is a *cause* for such and such health outcome. For example from the mere fact that lung cancer has a much higher incidence among smokers than among non-smokers we cannot conclude that smoking causes lung cancer in the usual sense of the expression "to cause". Nevertheless, we can exploit this fact in two ways. Firstly, we can plan and implement preventive measures as described in Sect. 2.3; see also Sect. 22.4. Secondly, epidemiologic observations and studies may prompt us to search for cause-effect relationships.

To stimulate an aetiological investigation, the purely epidemiologic knowledge obtained from appropriate studies may suffice; previous knowledge about causal mechanisms is usually not necessary.

The question of the aetiology of diseases is of course very old. It played an important role in medical writings in antiquity, both in China and in Europe. Many medical texts from and before the second century B.C. were found in Chinese graves, for example 15 texts in the Han tombs in Mavangdui in the province of Hunan. They present both the old ideas about evil spirits causing diseases and more modern theories about the role of environmental factors such as cold and heat, humidity and aridity and even microorganisms. The best-known presumed aetiological agent in Greece was that of a "*miasma*" (Greek: dirt) that was not laid to rest until the late nineteenth century. At that time the discussion was revived because microorganisms were discovered as causes of diseases; see Sect. 4.3. It led to the so-called "Henle-Koch postulates" for a pathogen to be the cause of a specific infectious disease. They are being treated in medical courses and will not be taken up here. They are also partly superseded since the contribution of other factors in addition to the infection itself has been investigated intensively; see again Sect. 4.3.

More recently the discussion around the meaning of the term "cause" and its place in epidemiology has taken new forms. Part of it is fairly abstract and we shall not pursue it here. A larger part, however, has arisen in connection with specific diseases, especially non-infectious ones like cancer, cardio-vascular diseases and diabetes. We shall have a look at it in the relevant sections and in Sects. 16.2 and 17.2.

15.4 Practical Work

1. Prove the relation given in Sect. 15.1 between prevalence, incidence and average duration of a disease, assuming that all cases have the same duration. Hint: Find the prevalence at time 0 by counting all cases that started at some moment before time 0 and still exist at that time. Reason first with a specific duration, for example three units of time.
2. Go back to the table in Sect. 10.3 and the first problem of Sect. 10.5, and try again to interpret the differences of the quotient "prevalence/incidence" between the various areas. Note that in view of the relation stated in Sect. 15.1, either the situation is not stable over time in some areas or the average duration of the disease HIV/AIDS is not the same in all areas, or both.
3. Draw the "curve of odds" $y = p/(1 - p)$ in the py-plane for $0 < p < 1$. Compare risk ratio and odds ratio for various values of the risks p and p' such as: $p = 0.003$, $p' = 0.001$; $p = 0.4$, $p' = 0.1$; $p = 0.999$, $p' = 0.99$.

Lesson 16
Cross-Sectional Studies

It is explained what a cross-sectional study is, when it should be performed and why.

16.1 Definition, Implementation and Evaluation

Cross-sectional studies are related to sample surveys. In both types of studies a sample S is taken from the target population U, for example by one of the sampling plans presented in Sect. 12.2. The basic difference between the two studies resides in their purpose and, consequently, in the way they are being evaluated. As remarked in Sect. 12.4 the purpose of a typical sample survey is to estimate indicators of variables *separately* for each variable of interest; in most surveys, these indicators have the form of a mean. For example in a household survey, we might want to estimate the average number of people in a household, the average income of a household, their average outlay for health care, their average number of consultations per year at their Commune Health Station etc.

By contrast, in a cross-sectional study we are mainly interested in *relations* between variables, especially between risk factors, also called exposures, on the one hand and health outcomes on the other hand. We may keep in mind the example from the second part of Sect. 15.1. Thus the target population U consists of all adult inhabitants of the province of Thai Binh on the 1st January 2016. The exposure variable takes two values, namely 1 for exposed subjects defined as those who had no secondary education on that date, and 0 for the other, non-exposed subjects. The outcome variable has the value 1 for diseased people, defined as those who suffer on the 1st January 2016 from pulmonary tuberculosis, and the value 0 for non-diseased people.

In a cross-sectional study the investigator usually estimates the risks p and p' in the target population directly by the corresponding risks $p_s = a/(a + b)$ and $p_s' = c/(c + d)$ in the study population. There exist several kinds of epidemiologic software that calculate these two estimated risks including confidence intervals. They calculate as well the estimator $r_s = p_s/p_s'$ of the risk ratio r and the estimator

© Springer Nature Switzerland AG 2019
K. Krickeberg et al., *Epidemiology*, Statistics for Biology and Health,
https://doi.org/10.1007/978-3-030-16368-6_16

$\eta_s = 1 - 1/r_s$ of the aetiological fraction among exposed with the corresponding confidence intervals. They also allow to test, for example, a hypothesis of the form H_1: $r > 1$, that is, the exposition has the effect of raising the prevalence, against the null hypothesis H_0: $r \leq 1$, on a given confidence level, or indicate the p-value of the data for these hypotheses.

These procedures rest on the following idea. Having selected the sample S independently of the exposure and of the outcome, the part of S that consists of its exposed subjects may be regarded as a sample S_1 from all exposed people and likewise for the sample S_0 of all non-exposed subjects in S. We then apply the methods described in the Lessons 12 and 14 for estimating a population proportion by a sample proportion and related inference.

However, the way we have obtained S_1 may not be a "good" sampling plan. In particular the size of S_1 is not fixed in advance in contrast to the size of a sample under the usual sampling plans. It depends on S and may be very small. It can also happen that we have only very few non-exposed persons in the sample S so that S_0 turns out to be small. The assumptions on which the methods described in Sects. 14.3 and 14.4 for evaluating the data in these samples rest, in particular approximate normality of the distribution of certain sample statistics, may not hold. Therefore, again:

When you intend to evaluate a cross-sectional study with the help of some ready-made statistical software, reflect on its inherent assumptions.

16.2   Advantages and Drawbacks of Cross-Sectional Studies

Let us start by citing again a truism: before embarking on any study the investigator needs to think carefully about which type of study can answer best the questions in which he or she is interested. Cross-sectional studies are frequent. Compared with most other types of epidemiologic studies, they are easier to plan and to implement. By their definition, they involve a single sample.

In most cross-sectional surveys the data are obtained, as in a sample survey, within a relatively short period of time immediately after taking the sample. Hence:

Most cross-sectional surveys make use of data that are available around the moment of drawing the sample.

The data may concern the present or the past. This happens in particular when the sample and the data are taken directly from existing registers; many cross-sectional studies are of this kind.

In other kinds of cross-sectional studies, the data are measured for the subjects in the sample at the moment of the study. Let us look at our example from this point of view. The outcome variable, namely the presence of pulmonary tuberculosis, concerns the moment of taking the sample around the 1st January 2016. It can be measured by questioning the persons in the sample directly. The exposure variable about education is also to be measured by an interview with people in the sample and it concerns the present as well.

From the preceding remarks and in particular from our example it is clear that:

Cross-sectional surveys are especially appropriate for dealing with the *prevalence* of diseases.

If we want to infer from a cross-sectional survey something about the *incidence* of disease or death in the past and if there are no registers available, we can sometimes question people about what they remember. This is frequently being done in primary health care surveys and is called "retrospective (or oral) diagnosis" or "retrospective (or oral) autopsy", respectively. They are based on symptoms to be remembered and therefore easily prone to errors.

While cross-sectional studies, especially register-based ones, are in general easy to implement, they suffer from two drawbacks. The first one is technical. We have already mentioned it in the preceding section; let us take it up again from a different point of view. We draw the sample S from the target population U but we base the estimation of the risks on two subsamples of S. The first one, S_1, consists of all exposed persons in S and is used for estimating the risk p among the exposed. Similarly, the set S_0 of all non-exposed persons in S serves to estimate p'. These subsamples are completely determined by S and we cannot control them separately. It may happen that one of them, for example S_1, turns out to be very small, that is, we may find very few exposed subjects in our study even though they are perhaps quite frequent in U and we have chosen a large sample S. In that case, the estimation of p by p_s based on S_1 could be very bad. In practice this means that the investigator should always check whether there are both sufficiently many exposed and sufficiently many non-exposed subjects in his sample.

The studies to be presented in later lessons, namely cohort- and case-control studies operate with two samples drawn independently of each other and thus avoid the technical obstacle just described.

The second disadvantage of cross-sectional studies concerns the type of problems to be handled and their interpretation. It results from the fact that we are dealing only with data that are available at the moment of taking the sample. Let us look again at our example. Suppose that the estimated risk ratio r is much larger than 1 and that perhaps we have been able to accept the hypothesis H_1: $r > 1$ on a reasonably high level of confidence such as 95%. Then we can affirm that there exists a certain statistical association between the lack of secondary education on the day of the study and pulmonary tuberculosis on the same day; its prevalence density is higher among those not having received secondary education. Can we now conclude or at least suspect that the exposure has had a *causal* effect on the outcome? To answer this question let us recall that:

A cause must precede its effect in time.

In our example as in all cross-sectional studies that are not register-based, both the exposure and the outcome status concern the present. However, the education of a person and the evolution of his or her tuberculosis leading to the present status may have taken place to a large extent during the *same* period of the past so that the exposure did *not* precede the outcome. It is even conceivable that a child did not get a secondary education *because* it suffered from tuberculosis; this would still lead to the same statistical association.

Sometimes, in order to investigate the evolution of a situation in time, one draws a sample from the target population and then measures the exposure and outcome variables at several successive moments, for example on the 1st January of every year. This is called a "longitudinal" study; it is a repeated cross-sectional study with the same sample of subjects. Unfortunately, some authors mean by "longitudinal study" a cohort study, which may cause confusion.

16.3   Practical Work

1. Plan, implement, and evaluate a small cross-sectional study, for example with the exposure- and outcome variables as above but only in a small region around you instead of an entire province.
2. Read and comment critically the report on a cross-sectional study that has appeared in the literature.

Lesson 17
Cohort Studies

It is explained what a cohort study is, when it should be performed, and why.

17.1   Definition, Implementation and Evaluation

A cohort study operates with several independent samples, one for each combination of levels of the exposure variables. Again we shall restrict ourselves to the simplest situation where we have only one binary exposure variable that differentiates between "exposed" (1) and "non-exposed" (0) and one binary outcome variable with the values "diseased" (1) and "non-diseased" (0). The term "diseased" may designate other health outcomes such as a missing tooth or death in a traffic accident.

For illustration, we shall use this time a historical cohort study that has played a crucial role in public health. In 1951, the British epidemiologists R. Doll and A.B. Hill chose as their target population U all British physicians who at that time did not suffer from lung cancer. They defined what they meant by "smoker" (exposed) and "non-smoker" (non-exposed). They then selected, via questionnaires, a sample S_1 from among the smokers and a sample S_0 from among the non-smokers in U; these were the "cohorts". They followed the two cohorts during 20 years and recorded the outcome variable with the values "died by lung cancer" (1) or "did not die by lung cancer" (0).

Let us take up the general situation. The purpose of the study at hand is to observe the appearance of the disease among the exposed and among the non-exposed and to compare the two. Therefore, as in the preceding example, the target population will contain only non-diseased subjects. Having drawn the samples S_1 and S_0 from the exposed and the non-exposed, respectively, the investigator can estimate the corresponding risks p and p' separately in each group by applying the methods of Lesson 12. Thus he estimates p by the proportion p_s of diseased people in S_1 and p' by the proportion p_s' of diseased people in S_0. This gives him his estimate $r_s = p_s/p_s'$ of the risk ratio r from which he derives the estimate of the aetiologic fraction among the exposed. There exist many kinds of statistical software to do these calculations including confidence intervals, tests of hypotheses, and p-values.

© Springer Nature Switzerland AG 2019

K. Krickeberg et al., *Epidemiology*, Statistics for Biology and Health,

https://doi.org/10.1007/978-3-030-16368-6_17

In the study by Doll and Hill "diseased" was to be interpreted as "died by lung cancer". They also distinguished many more types of exposure defined by various smoking habits. For the exposure "smoking 15–24 cigarettes per day", the estimated risk ratio was $r_s = 18$, hence the estimated aetiological fraction among exposed was $\eta_s = 0.944$. Thus, over 9 out of 10 deaths by lung cancer among these smokers could be said to be *due* to their smoking habit.

It is important to note that, apart from their smoking habits, exposed and non-exposed people probably did not differ much regarding other traits such as social standing or habits. Therefore, we can suppose that the two samples of exposed and non-exposed persons are more or less alike except for their exposure. This makes it unlikely that the different mortality in them is due to another factor but smoking. Using the terminology of Sect. 21.1 we should say that there is probably no confounding factor at work.

17.2   Advantages, Drawbacks and Practical Issues of Cohort Studies

The first advantage of cohort studies is of a mathematical-statistical nature, and in essence we have already described it in the preceding Sects. 16.2 and 17.1. Since the investigator draws a sample from both the exposed and the non-exposed, independently of each other, he can control their sizes and thus adjust them to the intended precision of the estimates of the two risks p and p', in contrast to a cross-sectional study where he may end up with very few exposed or very few non-exposed subjects in his study.

The following disadvantage of a cohort study is again due to purely mathematical-statistical facts:

A cohort study is not well suited for estimating *small risks* unless the samples are very large.

We have indeed noted in Sects. 12.5 and 14.2 that in order to estimate small proportions with a reasonable degree of precision we need large samples. In practice, small risks manifest themselves by very few diseased persons in the two samples. To obtain a sufficiently large number of diseased persons a very long follow-up of the cohorts may be necessary as in the historic example described in the preceding section. We shall see in Sect. 20.2, that this is one of the main reasons for using instead so-called case-control studies.

In contrast to cross-sectional studies:

A cohort study may be called for if the exposure is rare.

In this case the investigator can often still form a sufficiently large cohort of exposed persons, for example by including all or at least most of the exposed subjects of the target population.

Apart from these mathematical-statistical questions, when is a cohort study indicated? For which kind of problems and in particular for which kind of exposure and outcome variables may it be used?

Regarding the exposures, since the samples are drawn from the exposed and from the non-exposed subjects, the exposure must have been defined and known at the beginning of the study. Hence it must concern the past or the present. It can be measured, for example, by checking registers or, more frequently, via questionnaires as in the Doll and Hill study.

The outcome variable, too, may concern the past and be obtained from registers. In this case one would have a so-called "historical" cohort study; it is also called a "retrospective" cohort study. This type of study is in fact not uncommon.

Most cohort studies are "prospective", though, which means that one follows the two cohorts over a certain period of time and then measures for all of its members the outcome. In these studies the outcome concerns the future. One starts with non-diseased subjects and then records cases of the disease as they appear. Thus:

Cohort studies are particularly appropriate for dealing with *incidences* of diseases.

Up to now, we have tacitly assumed that the underlying target population had already been defined in a reasonable way, the only restriction being that it should not include already diseased people. However for a given problem a suitable choice of the target population is not always obvious. In the Doll and Hill study the target population that consisted of all British physicians who in 1951 did not suffer from lung cancer seemed to be a natural choice. It is likely that a similar study in most other parts of the British adult population would have yielded similar results.

Let us look at another example. In Vietnam there are many small ceramic factories where workers are painting and glazing pottery before it is being cooked. The workers often inhale fumes of the paints, in particular solvents; they will be called "exposed". We are interested in knowing whether this exposure has a negative influence on their health as expressed, for instance, by the outcome "appearance of bronchial disorders". Suppose we choose the target population "all inhabitants of the province of Thai Binh in the age group 16–50 on the 1st January 2009". The group of non-exposed people, that is, not working in the paint-shop of a ceramic factory, is then certainly quite different in many ways from that of all exposed persons. In particular it may include many persons whose general health is not sufficiently good to allow them to work in a factory. As a consequence, even when the exposure actually causes bronchial disorders there may be more bronchial disorders among the non-exposed than among the exposed subjects. This paradox is sometimes called the "healthy worker effect". In order to avoid it, we would have to restrict the target population to obtain that the group of non-exposed persons resembles the one of exposed people as much as possible, which is not easy. One might try to include in the target population only workers in ceramic factories who do not come into contact with fumes of paints, or workers in comparable factories of another kind. The problem can also be treated from the point of view of confounding factors (Sect. 21.1).

Further examples of cohort studies will appear in Sects. 22.2, 22.3, 23.2, 25.2 and 26.2.

Let us finally come back to the question of *causality*. A prospective cohort study may lead us to suspect a causal relationship between the exposure and the health outcome because here the putative cause precedes the effect. Still, like any other type of epidemiologic study, it can reveal only a statistical association between exposure and outcome.

Epidemiologists have formulated various criteria in addition to "the cause must precede the effect" that should be verified before affirming that a causal relation is likely to exist.

The first is the "strength" of the association. For example, an estimated risk ratio of $r_s = 1.03$ would not be very convincing evidence even when the study would allow to accept the hypothesis H_1: $r > 1$ on the confidence level of, say, 95%. The second criterion is "consistency". It means that different studies of the relationship ought to point in the same direction. Finally, beyond the purely epidemiologic context, the causal relationship in question must be "plausible" in view of known biologic mechanisms.

Smoking as a risk factor for lung cancer satisfies these criteria. However, they are still not sufficient to establish a causal relationship with certainty. Theoretical research around the problem of causality in health, accompanied by many debates, continues. In practice epidemiologic studies usually provide first evidence, which will then be supported by biologic investigations into the aetiology of such and such disease.

Summing up, prospective cohort studies are particularly suited for investigating the influence of an exposition on an outcome that will happen, and can be observed in the future, provided that the risks p and p' to be estimated are not too small. Their main drawback is that the two cohorts often need to be followed over a very long time span, which may be costly but also present technical problems. In particular, members of cohorts may drop out, that is, "get lost out of sight" or "get lost to follow-up". These technical problems will be discussed in Lesson 27.

17.3 Practical Work

1. Plan, implement, and evaluate a small cohort study of your choice, lasting not more than half a year and concerning the incidence of a disease or of death in a Vietnamese context. A suitable outcome would be the appearance of a disease that usually happens rapidly and frequently after the beginning of the observation, for example influenza or traffic accidents. Decide yourself about relevant exposures.

2. Read and comment critically the report on a cohort study that has appeared in the literature.

Lesson 18
Clinical (Therapeutic) Trials

Clinical trials evaluate the normal curative activity of physicians, which consists in trying to cure or to alleviate diseases of individual patients. They also evaluate measures applied to individuals in order to prevent disease or death. Thus the exposure factor to be studied is "treatment", either curative or preventive.

18.1 Trials of Curative Treatments

We start by recalling some facts from previous lessons. There, many examples of exposures have appeared such as genetic disposition, smoking, lack of education, poor hygiene, polluted water, crowded housing, malnutrition, use of contaminated needles by drug addicts, and unprotected sex; many more will be treated in later lessons. They all exist independently of the health system. They belong to the first four categories of risk factors listed in Sect. 1.5, that is genetic factors, environmental factors, life style, and social and economic conditions. The study of such risk factors is called "observational" or "analytic" epidemiology because one observes and analyzes already existing situations; see Sect. 15.3. Normally we are of course interested in the influence of factors that make the risk of disease, death etc. *increase* when their level increases. Hence, as explained in Sect. 2.3:

The main application of analytic epidemiology is *prevention* by lowering the level of risk factors. We might call this "hygiene" in a very broad and modern sense.

One speaks for instance about "mental hygiene"as already said in Sect. 2.3.

However, there are also factors that are *created* by the health system with the explicit purpose of influencing health. After all, the normal activity of a physician, nurse, traditional healer etc. is just that. They treat a sick person in order to cure or alleviate his or her disease. It is hoped that this activity will have a positive influence but as we all know it may have negative effects, too, or be completely inefficient. The purpose of clinical trials is to evaluate the effect of a well-defined

© Springer Nature Switzerland AG 2019
K. Krickeberg et al., *Epidemiology*, Statistics for Biology and Health,
https://doi.org/10.1007/978-3-030-16368-6_18

treatment on health in a given target population; it is the study of the factor "treatment" in the general sense of epidemiology. This factor belongs to the fifth category in our list in Sect. 1.5.

The study of the action of factors that do not already exist but are created and controlled by the health system is called "experimental epidemiology". In particular:

By a clinical trial, also called "therapeutic trial", we investigate the effect of a treatment on health in a given target population. Thus it is part of epidemiology.

In the present section we deal with *curative* treatments. Their evaluation has of course been part of medicine from ancient times on. The oldest and still widely applied reasoning runs like this: after having received the treatment the patient did get better, hence the treatment was effective. In a few cases of spectacular recovery this argument has some value but in most cases the obvious comment to be made is that the patient may have got better also without the treatment. Recovery might have been due to some other factors such as the natural healing power of his or her body or a change of the weather.

This comment reminds us that the essence of the evaluation of treatments is *comparison* as everywhere in epidemiology. Often the physician or healer who has successfully applied a treatment knows that in the past people suffering from the same disease who did not get his treatment did not recover so well. He concludes that the treatment was efficient. These untreated persons of the past are then called "historical controls". Such a reasoning has often given valuable information but suffers from a similar flaw as before: conditions may have changed in time and some other factors such as lower economic standards in the past may have been the main cause for the poor performance of the treatment on the historical controls.

In a modern clinical trial the group of people who obtain the treatment to be evaluated and the group of people with whom they are to be compared are constructed by clear and rigorous rules. This is why we talk of "controlled" trials. Let us look at the technical aspects.

We assume that the disease to be treated was rigorously defined; we shall call it the "target disease". Our target population U consists of people suffering from it. To have an example in mind we may recall the study described in Sect. 3.4 and regard as our target population all married Vietnamese women aged 18–49 who, during a certain period, are diagnosed in a hospital as suffering from a benign wound of the cervix.

Next we have to define the outcome variable "result of the treatment" in a rigorous and verifiable way. In common language it may mean "improvement" or "recovery" or "survival beyond a given period of time" or still another aspect of the evolution of the disease. In our example it means complete healing of the wound. Criteria defining the outcome are sometimes called "endpoints" of the study.

After that, we pass to the "exposure" variable, that is, the treatments to be compared. We shall restrict ourselves to two treatments T_1 and T_0. Often, T_0 simply means the absence of any treatment, or it may be an older treatment with which we would like to compare a new treatment T_1. Again, both require a precise definition. In our example, T_0 is the use of Laser CO_2 and T_1 is galvanocautery.

The idea of a trial is to compare the outcome in a group S_1 of subjects treated by T_1 with the outcome in a group S_0 of people treated by T_0. The construction of these two groups is one of the crucial elements of the trial.

First we draw a sample S from U, that is a sample of persons suffering from the target disease. S is the study population in our previous terminology but in the present context its members are usually called "subjects in the trial". The mechanism for obtaining S, in other words the sampling plan, will of course depend very much on the type of the target disease. Since the subjects in the trial suffer already from it they will normally come from a hospital, a health centre or a medical practice. Often they volunteer to participate in the trial, but then the sample S obtained may not be "typical" or "representative" of the target population; for example, volunteers may be healthier and stronger than people in the target population in general. We shall come back to these problems in Sect. 27.2.

Next we divide S into the two parts S_1 and S_0. It is clear that the construction of S_1 and S_0, that is the choice of the treatment T_1 or T_0 to be given to a patient in the trial, must be completely independent of any other factor that could also influence the outcome of the treatment. For example we should not treat by T_1 all patients entering the trial during a given week and then by T_0 all patients arriving during the following week; the weather has perhaps changed a lot from the first to the second week and this could have influenced the speed of recovery. Now, nobody knows all the factors that might act on the result of the treatment. Therefore, the only way to exclude a possible link between such a factor and the choice of the treatment is to execute this choice in a completely random fashion.

It could be done like this. Suppose that we have a list of all patients in the trial. We then prepare, with the help of a computer or a table of random numbers, a sequence of random digits 0 and 1, for example with 20 patients,

$$1\,0\,0\,0\,0\,1\,0\,1\,1\,0\,0\,0\,0\,1\,0\,0\,0\,1\,1\,0.$$

Accordingly the first patient will be treated by T_1, the next four by T_0, the sixth by T_1 etc. This method is easy to implement but has the drawback that the sizes of the groups S_1 and S_0 also depend on chance and cannot be fixed beforehand. In a large trial with many subjects this does not matter because the ratio of the sizes of S_1 and S_0 will be approximately equal to the ratio of the probabilities of 1 and 0 in the mechanism for constructing the sequence of random digits; in the example above, obtained from a table of random numbers, both probabilities were equal to 1/2. For smaller trials, other random mechanisms exist that yield groups of sizes given in advance.

Whatever the random mechanism used may be, a trial where the treatments are allotted at random will be called "randomized". Hence:

A randomized controlled clinical trial evaluates the effect of treatments by comparing them with each other in a controlled fashion. Hereby, the allotment of such and such treatment to a subject is determined by a random mechanism, independently of any other factor that might influence the outcome.

Choosing the sample S correctly and dividing it into the two treatment groups S_1 and S_0 by an appropriate random mechanism is still being neglected in many clinical trials; recall the discussion in Sect. 3.4.

The following step is the *evaluation* of the result of the treatment for each patient, in other words the measurement of the outcome variable for each person in the trial. In our example this means deciding, for every patient, whether the wound has healed or not. This is a fairly objective decision to be checked in a laboratory. In many other trials, though, it is a more subjective decision of the type "the patient feels better" or "he has completely recovered" or "his dyspnoea has become less serious" or another endpoint that involves the judgment of the patient or of the physician who does the evaluation. This judgment is easily influenced by the knowledge that the patient or physician may have about the treatment administered. Indeed if we ask the patient "do you feel better?" and if he knows that he was treated by a new drug, he may be more likely to reply "yes" than if he knew that he got the old type of drug. Likewise, a physician hoping that a new treatment will turn out to be superior will be more inclined to declare it successful in a patient who had received it than in one who had not.

Given this weakness of the human mind, clinical trials need to be "blinded" as far as possible.

A trial is called "blinded" or, more explicitly, "patient blinded" if the patient ignores to which treatment he or she was submitted. It is called "doubly blinded" if the physician who judges the result of the treatment in a patient also does not know what the treatment was.

For drug treatments, blinding is usually easy to achieve. If the control treatment is "no treatment at all", a "placebo" can be given. If two drug treatments are to be compared, the drugs need to be indistinguishable by shape, colour, taste etc. Even an acupuncture trial can be patient blinded as it was done in a recent large trial in Germany. Some surgical treatments, too, were blinded by a "sham treatment", namely "simulated surgery". In most treatments of the type surgery, radiotherapy, dietary interventions or gymnastics, blinding is more difficult or impossible.

Double-blinding is usually achieved by entrusting the evaluation of endpoints to a physician who was not involved in providing the treatment.

Finally, we arrive at the last stage, namely analyzing and evaluating the entire trial. Before talking about the methods, let us look back at what we have done so far. First, we have constructed two groups of subjects S_1 and S_0 in which the treatments T_1 and T_0, respectively, were applied. Then we have followed these two groups and recorded for every one of its members the value of the outcome variable "effect of the treatment". This amounts to regarding S_1 and S_0 as *cohorts* to be followed up. A clinical trial is indeed essentially a cohort study. The only difference resides in the fact that in an analytic cohort study the exposure variable, or "risk factor", to be analyzed exists already and we draw a cohort from "exposed" and another one from "non-exposed" people. In a clinical trial, we first construct the cohorts and then determine the exposure variable "treatment" accordingly.

It is therefore not surprising that the methods for analyzing clinical trials and those for analytic cohort studies are largely the same, including the software to be used.

They depend of course very much on the form of the outcome variable "effect of the treatment".

It would be futile to deal in this book with many types of particular analyses. In practice one has to look up the right method when a specific problem presents itself. To illustrate the basic ideas, we assume again that there are only two outcomes "cured" and "not cured". Instead of the "risks of falling ill" for exposed and for non-exposed people as in an analytic cohort study we shall now have to estimate the "probability of getting cured" among people treated by T_1, to be denoted by p, and the same among people treated by T_0, to be denoted by p'. We use the table of Sect. 15.2 exactly as we did for a cohort study in Sect. 17.1. This time we write a 2×2-table with the columns "cured" and "not-cured" and the rows "T_1" and "T_0". Thus a will be the number of subjects in the trial who had been treated by T_1 and were cured, etc. We can estimate p by $p_s = a/(a + b)$ and p' by $p_s' = c/(c + d)$, and we regard the quotient $r_s = p_s/p_s'$ as a good indicator for the efficacy of the treatment T_1 compared with T_0. For example, $r_s = 31$ would mean that, estimated on the basis of the trial, a person treated by T_1 has a 31 times larger probability of being cured than one treated by T_0. Normally we have to complement these estimations by calculating confidence intervals; sometimes we are also interested in a test of a hypothesis and a p-value. There exists of course software to do this easily.

In the example described in Sect. 3.4, the core of the final analysis is contained in the table there. The reader may draw the relevant conclusions himself or herself.

As noted in Sect. 17.2 this type of analysis supposes that neither p nor p' is very small since a precise estimation of small proportions requires large samples. If, for example, we get estimates $p_s = 0.97$ and $p_s' = 0.001$, we shall certainly not attempt to estimate the quotient $r = p/p'$. However it is still natural to consider these results as sufficient evidence for the superiority of the treatment T_1. We could calculate a confidence interval for p as further evidence.

18.2   Trials of Preventive Treatments

For *preventive* treatments the target population consists of healthy people, that is, persons who do not yet suffer from the "target" disease to be prevented. Otherwise, the principle of a trial is essentially the same as for a curative treatment. To be concrete, we shall describe it for a vaccine trial; we may think of a vaccination against hepatitis B as mentioned in Sect. 9.3.

First, we have to define the target population. It must consist of healthy persons and may be subject to further restrictions, for example comprising only people in a certain age group or only persons who have a particularly high risk of catching hepatitis B such as health personnel or injecting drug addicts.

The purpose of a trial is to evaluate the entire vaccination *procedure*, which is defined by the type of vaccine including dosage and the moment and method of administering it. The main component of the evaluation is the estimation of the efficacy η as defined in Sect. 5.3. Recall that it is the proportion of individuals who are *protected* by the vaccination among those who would have fallen ill if there had been no vaccination. This proportion depends of course on the "follow-up time", from the moment of the vaccination on, during which cases of the disease are observed and counted. The follow-up time is an indispensable component of the definition of η but unfortunately it is not always mentioned in presentations of a vaccine; we shall come back to this issue in Sect. 18.4.

To start the trial, the "persons in the trial" have to be selected, that is, the sample S needs to be constructed. The practical problems are similar to those sketched for curative trials. Often, one would like to involve in the trial *all* people of the target population in a given region and during a certain period but not all of them may agree to take part; this problem will be discussed further in Sect. 18.5. Sampling based on the recruitment of paid or unpaid volunteers may bring about a bias; see Sect. 27.2.

Next, the two "cohorts" S_1 of unvaccinated and S_0 of vaccinated people in S are constructed independently of any factor that could possibly exert an influence on the appearance of the disease. To this end, random mechanisms of the type described above for trials of curative treatments should be used.

Then we have to observe the two cohorts during the follow-up time. In order to evaluate the trial, the appearance or non-appearance of the disease in any person in the trial during this time has to be asserted. As in a trial of a curative treatment, this will normally require double blinding in order to assure objective diagnoses. Thus, neither the persons in the trial nor the physicians evaluating their health status must know whether a given subject had been vaccinated or not. A "placebo" vaccine can be used to this end.

Finally, in order to estimate the efficacy η we need to estimate the proportion p of diseased people among the unvaccinated and the proportion p' of diseased people among the vaccinated; recall that $\eta = (p - p')/p$.

Here we encounter the typical problems of cohort studies. Firstly, it may be necessary to follow the cohorts for a long time. For example, if we want to assert that the vaccination has an efficacy of, say, at least 80% over 10 years, the trial needs to last 10 years. Secondly, for most diseases the incidence during the trial period will be relatively small, which implies that the proportions p and p' will be small. Therefore, for a precise estimation large samples are required. The historic trial in the USA in 1954 of the Salk vaccine to prevent paralysis or death from poliomyelitis involved 1.8 million young children; the annual incidence rate of the disease before the trial was indeed only around 0.0005.

18.3   Further Thoughts

As said above, if a patient feels better after having received a specific treatment, we cannot conclude that it was due to the treatment. It may have been the result of another factor including the natural healing power of the human body.

Nowadays it seems obvious to all knowledgeable people in Public Health that a treatment can only be evaluated by comparing its results with those of other treatments, to be done by rigorous trials in well-defined populations. However, the history of medicine up to the present is full of widely applied therapies that finally turned out to be inefficient or harmful as eventually proven by a clinical trial. Thus in 1828 the French physician Pierre Charles Alexandre Louis published the result of one of the first carefully planned clinical trials ever performed. It showed that the century old practice of bloodletting by leeches, which had still been recommended shortly before against all kinds of inflammatory diseases, had in reality no effect at all. We shall not examine the long list of recent examples; it is certainly not closed.

The modern methods of clinical trials have been developed from the middle of the twentieth century on. It was also at that time that epidemiologists began insisting that in principle only therapies should be used in medicine that had been submitted to a rigorous evaluation of their efficacy, harmful side effects, and perhaps other characteristics such as a cost-benefit analysis. More recently, a movement was started under the name "Evidence-based Medicine" which has set itself the goal of promoting this idea systematically in medical practice. It is not always easy to do; we shall come back to the practical problems in the next section.

It is clear that *all* kinds of treatments in whatever framework should be judged by modern epidemiologic methods. In particular, in this regard there is no difference between "oriental" and "occidental" medicine. Performing more clinical trials in oriental medicine would certainly be very illuminating and useful. The same is true for the so-called "paramedical" activities in both oriental and occidental medicine, including those of traditional healers. Some may turn out to be useless but for others their efficacy may be confirmed.

All types of medicine (oriental, occidental, traditional, modern, "school" medicine, and paramedical) need to be evaluated by the same yardstick of controlled clinical trials.

Here are two examples of widely used treatments outside occidental school medicine. The first one is *acupuncture*. The large clinical trial mentioned in Sect. 18.1 and similar ones showed that, simply put, acupuncture is an efficient analgesic for some locations of pain but not for others. Second, there has never been a rigorous trial which could show that *homoeopathy* has any curative efficacy at all. In both examples patients may feel better after such a treatment by the placebo effect, which we have described in Sect. 18.1 in the context of "blinding" in a clinical trial.

18.4 Before and After a Clinical Trial

The trials whose basic principles we have sketched in Sects. 18.1 and 18.2 concern therapies that had already been rigorously defined. These trials evaluate such treatments in the target population where the treatments are to be applied in practice. They are therefore often called "field trials" and are based on epidemiologic principles and methods. They need to be distinguished from trials used in *developing* a new therapy. The latter are carried out in small populations constructed *ad hoc* and do not have much to do with epidemiology. We shall therefore sketch them only briefly, starting with the example of a hypothetical new curative drug therapy.

After initial studies in the laboratory and on animals there will be a "Phase I trial", which is largely pharmacologic. It concerns mainly the safety of the drug, in particular the dosage that can be administered without causing serious side effects. The efficacy of the drug is investigated for the first time in a "Phase II trial". Here, toxicity and side effects will be monitored again. It is in the Phase II trial that the form of the drug treatment to be finally submitted to a field trial, also called "Phase III trial", will be determined precisely. Often several "competing" drugs will be tested in parallel by Phase I and Phase II trials in order to select the one to be evaluated in Phase III.

Part of a Phase I trial can take place with healthy people but a Phase II trial requires patients. Both are usually done with volunteers. While a typical Phase I trial involves a few dozen subjects, a Phase II trial is usually larger, perhaps of the order of 100–200 patients.

For a preventive therapy, for example a vaccination, the Phase II trial faces a basic problem because in small study groups there will rarely be enough *potential* cases to be prevented; all subjects would have stayed healthy anyway even when not vaccinated. Sometimes, one resorts to a "challenge", that is, artificial infection of subjects by the target disease, which is of course a risky enterprise. In some countries, prisoners were used for this against a reduction of their term of imprisonment. Usually, however, the Phase II trial measures the effect of the vaccine only by its "immunogenicity", which is its capacity to provoke an immune response defined, for example, by amounts of antibodies. This is, however, not always indicative of the real efficacy in the sense of the capacity of preventing cases of the disease. The Phase III trial is therefore indispensable.

In most countries, new drug therapies and vaccines are only licensed for general use after trials of Phases I–III were performed and the results were considered satisfactory by the relevant health authorities. One flaw of this procedure is that the trials are mainly organized by the pharmaceutical companies which intend to sell these products and that their publications on the results are difficult to control and to evaluate. For example in the case of vaccine trials, the role of the length of time during which a given efficacy holds is often glossed over; see the discussion in Sect. 6.3 on Cholera and Rotavirus vaccines and Sect. 22.4 on the human papillomavirus.

A field trial, although done in the final target population, still takes place under controlled ideal conditions. These conditions may change once the treatment is being used routinely. In particular, due to material constraints and lack of training and motivation of the health personnel, the treatment may not be correctly applied and thus its efficacy may change, too; a break in the cool chain of a vaccine is a classical example. One therefore speaks of the "effectiveness" of the treatment under the conditions of normal practice. Measuring this effectiveness is sometimes called a "Phase IV trial".

The Phase IV trial also serves to monitor possible harmful side effects not yet discovered in previous trials. In fact:

For most modern treatments, especially by drugs, the problem of harmful side effects is at least as important as that of their efficacy.

This holds in particular for treatments of viral infections such as those by HIV, many forms of cancer, and cardio-vascular diseases. For example a largely applied drug treatment of arrhythmia has, in the long run, side effects that are in many respects worse than the condition treated.

A similar problem that often appears only in a Phase IV trial is that of the *interaction* of several medications, for example when taking at the same time a drug to strengthen the heart and one to treat an arrhythmia.

18.5   Ethical Issues

We have stressed the necessity of founding the routine treatments in medical practice on scientific evidence as provided mainly by rigorous clinical trials. We have, however, also encountered an "ethical" problem in such a trial, namely "challenges" in a Phase II vaccine trial. In Phase III trials, there is in principle *almost always* a fundamental ethical problem. For example, when starting a trial in order to compare two treatments T_1 and T_0 we usually have already some idea about the superiority of one of them, say T_1; this may be based on experiences in past practice or on a Phase II trial. The Phase III trial is then meant to confirm, or to refute, this idea. However, is it justifiable to give the treatment T_0, which we suspect to be inferior, to many people in the trial? The standard answer to this question is that as long as the inferiority of T_0 has not been established with certainty we are allowed to do it.

This ethical dilemma poses itself with more acuity in a curative drug trial when the drugs are to be taken over a long time, and also in a long-lasting vaccine trial. The superiority of a drug or a high efficacy of the vaccine may already become strikingly evident in a so-called "interim analysis" of the outcomes well before the intended end of the trial. May we then still continue the trial and withhold the seemingly better treatment from many subjects, or not vaccinate them?

The answers to these questions depend very much on the particular structure of a trial and have to be thought about very carefully in every case. There is, however, one rule that applies to all trials:

Every person to be recruited into a trial needs to be informed of its essential features, and needs to give what is called his or her "informed consent".

18.6   Practical Work

1. Organize a very simple trial to compare two curative treatments with a binary outcome that can be done in a district hospital, for example palliative treatments of the influenza syndrome.
2. Read and comment critically the report on a vaccine trial that has appeared in the literature, for example on vaccinations against rotavirus infections.

Lesson 19
Clinical Epidemiology

Clinical epidemiology is the application of epidemiologic knowledge to case-management and to related practice such as screening. Clinical trials are usually included but we have treated them separately in the preceding section because of their special weight in clinical practice.

19.1 Case-Management

A consultation in a Commune Health Station mostly runs like this:

Anamnesis, diagnosis, treatment.

This process is reflected by the layout of the Register of Consultations; see Sect. 11.1. It is the basic form of case-management. Normally the diagnosis is purely clinical and the resulting treatment is fairly standardized. The rules of the former programmes CDD (Control of Diarrhoeal Diseases; see Sects. 2.5 and 6.4) and ARI (Acute Respiratory Infections; see Sect. 2.5), now integrated in general clinical practice, provide good examples.

Sometimes the handling of a case in a Commune Health Station is more involved. There may be a follow-up or a transfer to another medical service. In a policlinic or hospital case management is often very complicated but the scheme above still forms its backbone. The two components "diagnosis, treatment" may no longer be separated conceptually, though. For example in medical services all over the world it is common to give antibiotics as soon as there is the slightest suspicion of an infection of any kind, bacterial or not. If it does not help, a bacterial infection is ruled out and there will be a more rigorous examination of the patient. In this way the treatment by antibiotics becomes *de facto* part of a differential diagnosis. For many diseases, even common ones like chronic bronchitis, the search for the cause by both diagnostic examinations and various treatments can go on in parallel for a long time. The case-management of tuberculosis, AIDS, cardiovascular diseases, cancer, diabetes and others may extend over long periods.

© Springer Nature Switzerland AG 2019
K. Krickeberg et al., *Epidemiology*, Statistics for Biology and Health,
https://doi.org/10.1007/978-3-030-16368-6_19

What is, then, the role of epidemiology in case-management? In a sense the answer is obvious. When a physician applies a diagnostic or therapeutic procedure he bases himself on knowledge about the properties of these procedures. This knowledge, however, had not been acquired by observing only a single case. It stems from observations in entire populations of patients. In the preceding lesson we have seen how the properties of treatments can be investigated by clinical trials, which concern the influence of the factor "treatment" on health. In the present lesson we shall learn how to define and to study characteristics of a diagnostic procedure, and we shall realize that diagnosis, too, is *formally* a factor that influences health. In both domains we are thus in the realm of epidemiology. Hence the answer to the question at the beginning of this paragraph will be:

Epidemiologic knowledge is used in every clinical act.

As before, in order to work out the basic ideas we shall restrict ourselves to very simple aspects of case-management.

19.2 Characteristics of a Diagnosis

In order to have something concrete in mind we may think about one of the following two classical diagnostic schemes. The first one is purely clinical and is sometimes used in Commune Health Stations to diagnose a case of shigellosis. According to this scheme a health worker or physician declares that the patient suffers from shigellosis if *all* the following signs are present:

1. Fever.
2. Diarrhoea.
3. Blood or mucus in the stool.

We shall call this a "positive" result of the diagnosis and denote it by T_+. If at least one of the three criteria above is not satisfied, the result of the diagnosis was "negative" and will be denoted by T_-. Of course the diagnosis T_+ may be wrong; the patient may have amoebic dysentery instead. Similarly, he or she may have shigellosis in spite of the diagnosis T_-. If he or she really suffers from shigellosis, we shall write D_+; if not, it will be indicated by D_-.

The second example is the Mantoux test for a past or present infection by tuberculosis. Again, we denote a positive result by T_+, a negative one by T_-, the actual existence of a past or present infection by D_+ and its absence by D_-.

To simplify the discussion we shall also call our diagnostic scheme for shigellosis a diagnostic, or medical, "test" although it is composed of three individual examinations.

For any subject, we obtain one of the following four constellations:

A true positive test: T_+ and D_+.
A false positive test: T_+ and D_-.

A false negative test: T_- and D_+.
A true negative test: T_- and D_-.

More precisely, we should talk here of a true positive *result* of the test etc., but the short expressions above are being widely used.

The characteristics of a diagnostic test concern a particular target population and are defined in terms of the frequency of the four constellations in it. In order to under-line the importance of a clear description of the target population, let us add a third example. Many years ago in remote areas of Cambodia where malaria was highly endemic, the following test was sometimes applied to start the case-management: A person who has fever and headache is supposed to suffer from malaria, and there-fore gets an anti-malaria drug immediately. In these areas the test was actually quite good and useful. This would certainly not be true in present day Thai Binh!

In our three examples above the target population consists of all subjects who, in a certain region and during a certain period, arrive at a Commune Health Station or hospital and are submitted to the diagnostic test in question because they are sus-pected of suffering from the target disease.

In order to convey to the reader the meaning of the *characteristics* of a diagnostic test we shall first state their definition in terms of probabilities. As in previous les-sons we shall not suppose the concepts of probability theory to be known; an intui-tive understanding is enough. We define:

The "sensitivity" of the test is the probability, among all subjects suffering from the disease, of a positive test, in short the probability of T_+ given D_+ .

Thus it is the probability of detecting the disease if the patient has really con-tracted it. For example when the test has the sensitivity $0.7 = 70\%$ and we select at random a group of diseased patients, about 70% of them should show a positive result of the test.

At first sight a high sensitivity of the test seems to be a highly desirable property. However, we must also make sure that we do not "detect" too many non-existing cases. For example the trivial test: "*Always* state that the patient has tuberculosis" has the highest sensitivity possible, namely $1 = 100\%$, but it is obviously useless.

Hence the definition of the "specificity" of the test:

The specificity of the test is the probability, among all subjects *not* suffering from the disease, of a negative test, in short the probability of T_- given D_-.

A high specificity contributes to preventing a superfluous treatment of healthy patients. We shall see below how we may have to "balance" sensitivity against specificity when actually constructing diagnostic tests. A high sensitivity often entails a low specificity and conversely.

These two characteristics of a test are particularly suited in a target population and a clinical situation where the physician is dealing with patients whom he already suspects of having attracted the disease. In screening programmes where he wants to discover cases in a relatively large population the following two characteristics are also of interest; they are called "predictive values".

The "**predictive value of a positive test" is the probability, among all sub-jects for which the test was positive, that the subject actually suffers from the disease, in short the probability of D_+ given T_+.**

Likewise the "predictive value of a negative test" is the probability, among all subjects for which the test was negative, that the subject does in fact not suffer from the disease, in short the probability of D_- given T_-.

There is an important difference between these two groups of characteristics of a test. In a target population of a well-determined type, for example a certain age group, the sensitivity and specificity do not depend on the frequency of the underlying disease. For the same test, they will be the same in two different regions or in two different clinics even though the disease may be very frequent in one of them and rare in the other. This allows us to use the same test everywhere. Predictive values, however, depend on the frequency of the target disease.

The definitions given above in terms of probabilities convey well the meaning of the four characteristics, but how do things look in practice? To see this, let us as imagine that we have a sample of n subjects from the target population and that we know, for all of them, *both* the real disease status and the result of the test. We can then make a 2×2-table analogous to Table 15.1, to be denoted Table 19.1.

It is very important, though, to realize that, as in all epidemiologic studies, the analysis and interpretation of such a table depends crucially on the way the sample and the data were obtained. If we have drawn, independently of each other, a sample of diseased persons and another one of non-diseased persons, we can *estimate* the sensitivity of the test by $a/(a + c)$ and its specificity by $d/(b + d)$ and even give con-fidence bounds. This means handling the study like a *case-control* study: the dis-eased persons are the cases and the non-diseased ones the controls. For more details, see Lesson 20.

If, however, we want to estimate predictive values, we have to draw independent samples of people featuring a positive result of the test and of people with a negative result. We then estimate the predictive value of a positive test by $a/(a + b)$ and the predictive value of a negative test by $d/(c + d)$. This amounts formally to a *cohort study*: the cohorts are composed of people having a positive and a negative test, respectively.

Such studies are to be conducted before the test is introduced into practice. When estimating for example the sensitivity of the test and drawing to this end a sample of diseased persons by an appropriate sampling plan, their *real* disease status, which is called the "gold standard", must of course be established with certainty by means that are independent of the test to be evaluated. This is normally done by more refined and thorough laboratory examinations, which would not be performed in

Table 19.1 Disease status (D) and test result (T)

	D_+	D_-	Total
T_+	a	b	$a + b$
T_-	c	d	$c + d$
Total	$a + c$	$b + d$	n

daily practice because they are too long or too expensive. The role of the test in practice is precisely to replace them, or at least to give quick first information.

It is illuminating to look at the evaluation of a diagnostic test in the context of primary health care under difficult conditions as in our third example above. There, health workers employed the test:

Declare that the patient has malaria if he suffers from headache and fever.

Its sensitivity is no doubt high but in order to know how many superfluous drug treatments will be performed we are interested in its specificity. As we have seen this requires a sample of persons of whom we are *certain* that they are free of malaria. Now, even in a fairly rudimentary system of primary health care, suspected malaria patients are usually being followed up and the resulting data are being recorded in registers. Hence, *in the long run*, it will be known for almost every one of them whether he or she actually had malaria or not. We can therefore take a sample of non-diseased persons from the register and estimate the specificity by $d/(b + d)$ where b is the number of subjects in the sample who had had a positive test result and d the number of those who had had a negative result, that is, no headache or no fever. This would be a "retrospective register-based study". It employs the method of "sampling from registers", which we have already met in Sect. 12.1. Unfortunately it is an underutilized method. Many expensive sample surveys are being carried out whose results could have been obtained cheaply from registers.

The tests in our three examples are "binary" by their very nature, that is, their result is either "positive" or "negative". Many other tests are based on a measurement whose result is a number, say ρ. The test result is called "positive" if ρ is "large" and "negative" if ρ is "small". In order to give a precise meaning to this, we need to fix a so-called "threshold value "τ and consider the result positive if $\rho > \tau$ and negative if $\rho \leq \tau$. The test which we have defined in this way depends on the threshold τ; thus there is a whole family of tests, namely one for every τ. It is clear that their sensitivity increases and their specificity decreases when we choose a smaller threshold τ; the opposite is true when we augment the threshold.

We can represent their behaviour graphically by the so-called "operating characteristics" where the sensitivity and specificity are drawn as functions of τ. This makes it easy to select a threshold, which provides a "balance" between the two that is regarded desirable in view of the health situation at hand. The curves in Fig. 19.1 were constructed artificially for better illustration. We see that for the threshold $\tau = 0.17$ we get a test whose sensitivity is roughly 0.63 and whose specificity is about 0.48.

Tests based on threshold values function in the same way as those based on reference values; see the example in Sect. 13.2.

Often, a diagnosis is based on the results of many diagnostic tests together as in our first example regarding shigellosis. One has tried to simplify complicated procedures by a "computer-aided diagnosis" where the computer derives the diagnosis from the available clinical symptoms and laboratory measurements. The basis of this procedure, stored in the computer, consists of the results of analyzing many previously observed cases. In order to estimate the characteristics of such a diagnostic

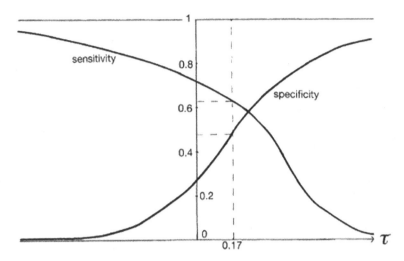

Fig. 19.1 An operating characteristics

scheme sufficiently well one needs to observe a relatively large number of cases. More powerful computing techniques allow some times to include the results of a very large number of cases into the basis of the procedure by observing them in extended areas of the world and in many countries. This is being considered somewhat pompously an "application of artificial intelligence". Deciding on the nature of an irregularity of the skin is a good example: benign or not, melanoma or not, nevus (beauty mark) etc. A recent diagnostic procedure uses the results of analyzing about 100,000 previous cases.

To conclude, let us ask whether we can really regard a diagnosis as a "factor" in the sense of the definition of epidemiology in Sect. 1.3 and claim that this factor "influences" health? The answer is easy if we recall that the epidemiologic concept of influence is purely statistical. Among people for whom the test was positive, the prevalence density of the target disease will in general not be the same as among people with a negative result; one would hope that it is higher because otherwise the test would not be very useful! It is this difference between the two prevalence densities that represents the influence of the factor "diagnosis".

19.3   Screening

We have already treated this topic briefly in Sect. 2.4. Let us take it up again in the light of what we have learned in the mean time. We start with a slightly shorter definition:

Screening is the systematic search for cases of a disease that have not yet declared themselves, in short: early detection.

Its purpose is twofold:

- To treat the cases found at an early stage when the chance of curing them is still higher. Thus the existence of a helpful early treatment is an essential condition for embarking on screening.
- For an infectious disease, to reduce the number of potential sources of infection by an early treatment or by isolation of the patients found.

Screening is, in the first place, a diagnostic activity. Since it serves to prevent existing cases from passing to a stage where they can no longer be treated successfully, it is also called "secondary prevention".

Screening has a long tradition. In a less systematic form it was done for leprosy already in antiquity. In many countries screening has been the centrepiece of medical care in schools; see Sect. 2.4. For a long time screening for pulmonary tuberculosis was widely done by X-rays, the Mantoux test or a sputum examination; see Sect. 7.3. In a sense, active case finding, for example of malaria within primary health care, is a screening activity and so is the systematic follow-up of mother and child within the MCH (Mother and Child Health) programme.

More recent screening programmes concern breast cancer and cervical cancer of women, prostate cancer of men (Sect. 22.4) and HIV-infections (Sects. 10.2 and 10.5).

The first step to be taken when setting up a screening programme is to define the target population which is also called the "screened population". In schools one needs to decide whether to examine only children in their first year of school or also those in higher grades. Very often, screening will be restricted to high-risk groups. For example in France until a few decades ago, all employed people had to undergo a yearly X-ray examination in view of early detection of pulmonary tuberculosis, but now only small high-risk groups are being screened systematically. For cancer of the colon, typical high-risk people are those with antecedents of polyps in the colon. Risk groups for HIV-infections are well known; see Lesson 10.

Next, we need to select the test to be used. Often, for example for tuberculosis, we have the choice between several ones. Cost and technical constraints will play an important role but the main criteria will be the four characteristics of the tests to choose from. In particular, recall that their sensitivity and specificity do not depend on the frequency of the target disease. The predictive value of a positive test, however, will become smaller if the prevalence of the disease decreases; thus the percentage of actual cases among subjects with a positive test result will then also be smaller, and analogously for negative results.

Let us illustrate this by screening for an HIV-infection. There are tests meant to discover antibodies (seroconversion) and others that show the presence of the virus itself in serum, saliva or sputum. The first ones are rapid and cheap and have a high sensitivity but low specificity; their objective is to find "suspected" cases. In Vietnam, the so-called "particle agglutination test SERODIA" is widely being applied for that. Then, among suspected subjects, a test of high specificity such as Western Blot can be used for confirmation of the infection.

At first sight, the idea of screening looks seducing. Saving lives or improving the quality of life for many years by early treatment seems to be excellent. However, there are many aspects to be taken into account before setting up a screening programme, and some programmes that have been going on for a while are the subject of heated discussions about their merits and flaws. They concern in particular:

- The "balance" between sensitivity and specificity. A *high* sensitivity is desirable in order to detect most existing cases but it generally entails a low specificity, that is, many false positive results. Such results can have serious consequences. The subjects will be alarmed for nothing. They may even be treated without further careful examinations for non-existing cases. This has been happening for example in prostate cancer screening by the search for PSA (prostate-specific antigen).
- "Over-diagnosis", for example of prostate cancer. It means surgery or radiotherapy of existing but light cases that would not have hurt the subject much if they had been left untreated. It entails needless suffering including impotency and incontinency.
- *Low* sensitivity: Taking part in the programme and having had no positive test results may reassure the subjects and thereby reduce their vigilance.
- Harmful side effects of the tests, for example of those using X-rays.
- Cost and benefits: it may very well happen that the money spent would have brought higher benefits if invested in other, especially preventive, measures, for example good health education.
- The benefit of the programme depends much on which members of the intended screening population actually take part in it. Often it is the healthier people and people of a higher socio-economic standing who are more likely to submit to the tests that are being offered.

Thus, careful deliberations by health authorities are necessary before starting a screening programme. They should be objective, which means in particular not be influenced by producers of equipment such as X-ray apparatus. The existence of a "helpful" treatment of early stages is essential; the treatment ought to improve the prognosis. The recommended frequency of testing needs to be defined; it depends on the "normal" course of the disease without screening. There is no use screening for a target disease that is rare or not very serious.

Each screening programme that has been going on for a while ought to be evaluated. We shall not deal with this aspect except in the specific context of cancer epidemiology; see Sect. 22.4.

19.4   Decision Rules

When reviewing textbooks on clinical epidemiology one discovers that there is no general agreement on what this field comprises. The simple definition given at the beginning of this lesson seems to be preferable from both a theoretical and a practical point of view. To conclude our round through this field we shall go back to everyday case-management. In order to simplify the picture we shall assume that all physicians and health workers are female and all patients are male.

There are situations where the course of action is in principle rigorously determined. Dehydration of children due to diarrhoea is a typical example; see Sect. 6.4. According to the CDD-rules the health worker or physician follows a strict decision scheme. First, on the basis of the anamnesis and a few well-defined clinical symptoms, the diagnosis is stated in the form of an unambiguously defined degree of dehydration. This degree alone determines the treatment. Similar strict decision rules govern procedures within the programmes ARI (Acute Respiratory Infections) and MCH (Mother and Child Health).

These rules have of course been established on the basis of epidemiologic investigations, in particular clinical trials and studies of the diagnostic tests used, so as to provide maximum benefit. They play an important role in primary health care because even health workers who have not received advanced medical training can apply them. For a full-fledged physician they make it easier to reach quick decisions.

Normally, however, the physician who is facing a patient has the choice between several options and needs to take decisions of her own. The question arises on which elements she should base them. In practice she decides according to her own good judgement, her knowledge of the properties of various diagnostic procedures and of the effects of the possible treatments available to her. However, there is also a theory called "medical decision analysis" that attempts to deal with this problem in a systematic way. We are going to present its basic ideas with the help of an example, namely the handling of cardiovascular diseases, described in a very simplified way.

Case-management of a cardiovascular disease is usually a long chain of stages and decisions. We shall distinguish decisions of the physician and decisions of "nature"; the latter may for example be "the patient recovers". At a given stage, the physician has the choice between two decisions:

P_1: Give the patient drugs and send him home.
P_2: Hospitalize the patient for diagnostic tests and treatment.

Then, nature can take one of the following two decisions:

D_1: The patient recovers.
D_2: He stays ill.

Each possible chain of events, that is, of decisions of the physician and of nature, can be represented by a "branch", or "path", in a "decision tree" like the one in Fig. 19.2.

Here decisions taken by the physician are represented by the symbol $\otimes$, those by nature by the symbol $\oplus$ and R is the end of a path due to recovery of the patient; C means "continue!" In the particular path drawn as a heavy line, the following events have taken place: The physician has hospitalized the patient after a first diagnosis (P_2). The patient was not cured (D_2). The physician then sends him home and prescribes a drug treatment (P_1). The patient still does not recover (D_2).

Now the physician has to decide about her next action. What are the elements on which she should base this decision? In principle, she should exploit the following knowledge:

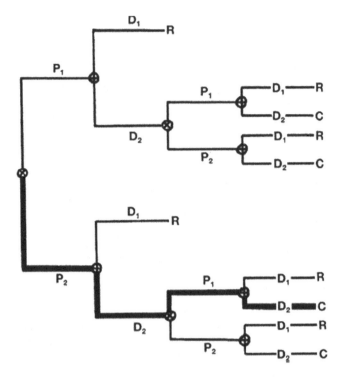

Fig. 19.2 A decision tree

- For each of the two possible decisions open her, the probability that they will result in the recovery of the patient.

For the decision of the physician at this stage and the decision of nature at the next one, there are four possible outcomes: D_1P_1 (drug treatment at home and recovery), D_1P_2, D_2P_1 and D_2P_2. The decision of the physician should also depend on the following elements:

- The "benefit" or "harm" due to any of these four possible outcomes.

The benefit or harm is represented by numbers, which are called "scores". A benefit may be a complete cure, higher life expectancy, better quality of life etc. Harm may mean side effects of the treatment such as toxicity, loss of some body functions due to surgery and others. Scores also take into account the cost of the two possible decisions of the physician, that is, of a drug treatment at home or another, perhaps expensive, stay in the hospital with more examinations, follow-up etc.

Given scores and the probability of outcomes, the physician will reach her decision by abiding to the following rule, which underlies in principle all of clinical epidemiology:

In case-management, given all the information available, in particular epidemiologic knowledge, the physician decides so as to maximize the expected benefit.

We shall not give here a rigorous definition of an "expected" benefit. Its intuitive meaning as an "average" benefit should be clear.

In practice, complicated decision rules are hardly ever applied. One of the main reasons is the difficulty in determining scores. Scores need to be based as much as possible not only on the subjective assessment by the physician involved but also on past experiences by the medical community and, in the ideal case, on previous rigorous studies, but in fact they remain fairly arbitrary. Therefore even large computer programmes are not very helpful. It may sound surprising at first sight but it is true that decision rules play their main role in *primary health care* and not on a higher level.

Scores depend on the *prognosis* of the case at a given moment when we know its previous history and the decisions of the physician. This would lead us to another part of clinical epidemiology, namely "prognostic medicine". We shall not treat it here; see, however, the related topic of "Genetic Prediction" in Sect. 26.4.

19.5 Practical Work

1. Organize a small study to find the four characteristics of a test that is commonly being used in primary health care.
2. Study and describe the screening programmes in Vietnamese schools.
3. Try to extract decision rules that are being applied in Mother and Child Health (MCH) and formulate them precisely.

Lesson 20
Case–Control Studies

It is explained what a case–control study is, when it should be performed, and why.

20.1 Definition, Implementation and Evaluation

In the following discussion we remain in the simple setting of Sect. 15.2, namely that of a single binary risk factor with the values "exposed" and "not exposed", and a binary outcome variable with the values "diseased" and "not diseased". We suggest that the gentle reader take another look at the discussion in Sect. 13.4 of the two ways of analyzing a 2×2–Table and in Sect. 15.2 of the basic concepts underlying epidemiologic studies.

Until now we have mainly treated cohort studies. This was true for analytic studies conducted by following up certain cohorts in order to investigate the influence of a risk factor on health. It was equally true for clinical trials. It also holds for the estimation of the predictive values of a diagnostic test where we start from two "cohorts", namely people with a positive test result on the one hand and those with a negative result on the other.

However, cohort studies face various problems as we have seen in Sect. 17.2. In an analytic cohort study of a rare disease only few cases may appear in the two cohorts even after we have followed them for a long time. This results in large errors in the estimation of the risks and the relative risk, and in high cost. Hence the idea of a quicker and more precise type of study came up where we *begin* by procuring us sufficiently many cases, for example from hospitals.

In a case-control study we do not compare, as in a cohort study, two groups of subjects defined by two different levels of the risk factor, but two groups determined by two different levels of the outcome variable, namely a group of "cases" and a group of "controls".

The idea of a case–control study has already appeared in Sect. 3.2. Before embarking on a general discussion we shall present another example in order to illustrate various aspects. This study was conducted in a gynaecologic hospital of

© Springer Nature Switzerland AG 2019
K. Krickeberg et al., *Epidemiology*, Statistics for Biology and Health,
https://doi.org/10.1007/978-3-030-16368-6_20

Ho Chi Minh-City. Its objective was to investigate risk factors for osteoporosis among postmenopausal women. Osteoporosis was defined by low bone mineral density, not to be made precise here. Several risk factors were considered such as low body weight (<44 kg) and corticosteroid treatment of arthritis; let us first fix our attention on one of them.

We shall first sketch the principle of the evaluation of a study and then look into the practical aspects of its implementation.

As always, we assume that we are dealing with a well-defined target population U. In our example we define it to be the set of all women living in the year 2007 in Ho Chi Minh-City whose menopause started at least 2 years ago. We draw a sample S^1 of cases of the disease and also select from U a sample S^0 of subjects who are not diseased; the latter are called "controls". These two samples need to be constructed independently of the risk factor to be studied; we shall come back later to the practical aspects of their construction. The two samples S^1 and S^0 together form the study population.

Next, for each subject in the samples we measure the risk factor, that is we find out whether the subject was exposed or not. Thus we get again a table as in Sect. 15.2. Its evaluation, however, will be different from the evaluation of a cohort study. The risks p_s and p_s' in the study population are indeed unsuitable for estimating the risks p and p' among exposed and non-exposed subjects in the target population U and likewise the risk ratio r_s in the study population may be very far from the risk ratio r in U. It can easily be proved, though, that the "odds ratio"

$$q_s = \frac{ad}{bc}$$

in the study population is a suitable estimator of the odds ratio q in the target population. The meaning of "suitable" for an estimator in the present context is essentially the same as in Sect. 14.3. It also depends on the way the controls are defined: see below. At any rate every common epidemiologic software will compute the estimator and confidence bounds for q as a function of the data. Recall from Lesson 14 that they are usually based on certain approximations using the normal law.

But what is the use of having estimated an odds ratio? We have already answered this question in Sect. 15.1. Sometimes one may just find it interesting to compare the odds among exposed and non-exposed people. One may also have in mind that $1 < q$ if and only if $1 < r$, that is if the factor is likely to increase the prevalence of the disease. However, in most applications the ultimate goal is still to estimate the risk ratio in the target population because this is what is usually needed in public health planning. In such a setting the odds ratio is mainly useful for the study of rare diseases because of the following simple but fundamental fact that we have made precise in the form of (15.1) of Sect. 15.1:

For a rare disease, the odds ratio is close to the risk ratio.

Having sketched the basic ideas of the numerical evaluation of a case–control study, let us return briefly to the stage before, namely the implementation. The essential step is of course the construction of the two samples. In most studies, the *cases* that form the sample S^1 come from health stations, policlinics, and hospitals. The registers of these health institutions may be helpful there, and so may be, for example, a central cancer registry. Sometimes it will be possible to include into S^1 *all* cases that have occurred in the target population U during the underlying period; this is of course the ideal situation. In any event, S^1 ought to be representative of the set of all cases in U in the sense of sampling theory. This is not guaranteed automatically if we take only cases from health stations and hospitals while U extends beyond that. If, for example, U consists of all inhabitants of a district, it is conceivable that very poor diseased people or diseased people living in remote areas do not seek treatment and are therefore underrepresented in S^1. This would be a form of the so-called "hospital bias"; see Sect. 27.2 for further discussion.

Constructing a sufficiently large good sample of *controls* S^0 is usually even more difficult. In older studies they were frequently selected from patients who had been hospitalized in the same institution as the cases but for another illness. Such a sample, too, is of course afflicted by hospital bias; it is rarely representative of the set of all non-diseased persons of the target population.

For a correct evaluation as sketched above we need to obtain a sample S^0 that distinguishes itself from S^1 only by the disease status but not by any factor that might be connected with the risk factor to be studied. A way to do this is to select S^0 from *all* non-cases of the target population U by a correct sampling plan. However, this is frequently unpractical or even impossible. Instead, a different scheme is often used. We construct the controls by what is called "matching". For each case, we select a few controls, usually 1, 2 or 3, who resemble the case in all aspects, which in our eyes might possibly influence the risk factor under scrutiny. We omit the technical details of the statistical evaluation for such a matched study.

In the study of risk factors for osteoporosis among women in menopause, the sample S^1 of cases consisted of 224 women taken from a gynaecologic hospital in Ho Chi Minh-City. Then 244 controls were obtained by matching. For each case, one or several women of the target population were selected who did not suffer from osteoporosis and resembled the case regarding the main personal, economic, and social characteristics.

In this study, it was easy to measure the exposures of the cases and controls. When looking at the factor "low weight", an estimated odds ratio of 3.6 was found with a confidence interval [1.1; 15.4] on the level 95%. For the factor "corticosteroid treatment" the estimated odds ratio was 2.9 with a corresponding confidence interval [1.5; 6.2]. As everywhere in the world, the prevalence of osteoporosis is not well known in Ho Chi Minh-City, but it is no doubt not very low. Hence we cannot derive from these odds ratios good estimates of the corresponding relative risks.

20.2 Discussion, Applications

Case–control studies are practically always analytic, that is, observational. Their goal is to analyze the influence of a risk factor. We start from cases and controls and then measure their exposure. Exposures have happened in the past or are happening at present. Thus a case-control study is necessarily *retrospective*. It can be used for a first investigation into a causal relation. Recall, however, from Sect. 17.2 that a cohort study, too, may be retrospective (historical).

The main advantages of a case–control study have already been briefly mentioned.

Firstly, we can obtain sufficiently many cases to ensure reasonably precise estimations.

Secondly, no long follow-up is required; a case–control study can generally be done in a relatively short time and is cheaper.

However, case–control studies also suffer from practical difficulties and basic drawbacks.

Firstly, exposures of cases and controls concern the past and are therefore often difficult to measure. The variables recorded in registers, such as sex and age are rarely those that form the subject of the study; even personal health cards, if they exist, contain only a few basic exposure variables. To measure a typical exposure like smoking habits or the consumption of alcohol in the past, one has to resort to questionnaires that are given to all subjects of the study population. The answers may not be reliable for various reasons, in particular failing memory or reluctance to admit bad habits. Other types of past exposures, especially socio-economic ones such as profession or housing conditions may be easier to measure.

Secondly, as explained above, it is often hard to build a good sample of controls.

Thirdly, only the odds ratio but not the risk ratio can be estimated from a case–control study. For diseases that are not too frequent we will approximate the risk ratio by the odds ratio but a case–control study of an epidemic of seasonal influenza would hardly yield useful insights!

Lastly, if the exposition or the absence of the exposition is rare, the estimate of the odds ratio might be very imprecise.

Applications of case–control studies will appear in later lessons, namely in Sects. 22.2, 22.3, 25.3, and 26.3. In addition, we are going to sketch two more categories of applications.

The first category is very old. It consists of outbreak investigations of infectious diseases; see Sects. 3.2 and 4.5. The principle is simple: look at the cases that were found; take a few controls; try to discover expositions that are much more present among cases than among controls. The investigation of food poisonings is a classical example; we may think of the presence of Salmonella as the exposure.

A second category of applications concerns the effect of a preventive measure when the health outcome to be prevented is rare. For example in a Mother and Child Health programme the health outcome may mean "maternal death" and the exposition may be "not having attended the prenatal examinations that were foreseen".

20.3 Practical Work

1. Plan, implement, and evaluate a small case–control study of your choice in a Commune Health Station.
2. Write a plan how to conduct a study on maternal mortality as sketched above. In particular, describe in precise terms the target population, the exposure, the outcome, samples to be taken, and the evaluation. Is it possible to estimate a risk ratio?
3. Read, and comment critically, the report on a case–control study that has appeared in the literature.

Lesson 21
Confounding

The influence of a risk factor as found in a study may be only apparent and reflect the influence of another factor with which it is connected.

21.1 The Idea of Confounding in an Example

Up to now we have been studying the influence of a *single* factor on the distribution of a disease or of other health-related characteristics. This allowed us to concentrate on the essential ideas. Most diseases are "multi-factorial", though; many factors exert their influence together. In this book we shall not deal with general methods that have been developed in order to analyze their joint influence; some tools will be mentioned in Lesson 28. The present lesson is devoted to a different problem, namely that of a factor which "confounds" the action of another one. It is of utmost importance.

Let us go back to the example presented in Sect. 15.1, which is about the influence of the factor "education" on the prevalence of pulmonary tuberculosis. Suppose that in a study we have found a much higher prevalence among the "exposed" subjects, who are those who had only primary education, than among people having obtained secondary education. Can we conclude that education influences tuberculosis directly, perhaps even in the sense of a causal relationship?

If we look back at the long history of tuberculosis as sketched in Sect. 7.1, we see that other factors have been incriminated in addition to education, in particular housing; crowded housing favours indeed mutual infections. Perhaps the factors "education" and "housing" are somehow related with each other? For example if among people with only primary education, poor housing is more frequent than among people with secondary education, and if it is poor housing that raises the prevalence of pulmonary tuberculosis significantly, then a study would also show an influence of education on the disease even while there was no causal influence at all. How can we disentangle these actions by purely epidemiologic, statistical, methods?

Let us investigate a fictitious particular situation. The target population consists of 200 people and the cases are distributed in it according to Table 21.1.

© Springer Nature Switzerland AG 2019
K. Krickeberg et al., *Epidemiology*, Statistics for Biology and Health,
https://doi.org/10.1007/978-3-030-16368-6_21

We note that the prevalence of tuberculosis in the whole population is 40, hence the prevalence density is 40/200 = 0.2 = 20%.

The influence of the factor "education" can be calculated from the following Table 21.2, which we derive from Table 21.1. Thus, the risk of tuberculosis among subjects with only primary education is 28/100 = 0.28 and among those with secondary education it is 12/100 = 0.12; hence the risk ratio for the factor "education" is 28/12 ≈ 2.33. Similarly, for the factor "housing" we have Table 21.3.

This furnishes the risk 0.3 given poor housing and 0.1 given good housing, hence a risk ratio of 3.

The two risk factors are obviously linked. 90% of people with only primary education live in poor housing conditions but only 10% of those who have received secondary education do.

We shall now examine the influence of the factor "education" separately among people in poor housing conditions on the one hand and among those in good housing conditions on the other hand. We call this "controlling" for the factor housing when investigating the action of the factor education. First we look at subjects living in poor housing conditions. In this population the risk of tuberculosis is 27/90 = 0.3 among people with only primary education and 3/10 = 0.3 among people with secondary education, which results in the risk ratio 1. The same is true in the population that consists of all people in good housing conditions. Indeed, there the risk among people with only primary education is 1/10 = 0.1 and among people with secondary education it is 9/90 = 0.1, hence again a risk ratio 1. Thus in these two subpopulations defined by a same housing standard, the factor education has no influence at all!

This leads us to the following general definition:

Table 21.1 Prevalence of pulmonary tuberculosis by education and housing

Education	Housing	Diseased	Not diseased	Total
Only primary	Poor	27	63	90
Only primary	Good	1	9	10
Secondary	Poor	3	7	10
Secondary	Good	9	81	90

Table 21.2 Prevalence of pulmonary tuberculosis by education

Education	Diseased	Not diseased	Total
Only primary	28	72	100
Secondary	12	88	100

Table 21.3 Prevalence of pulmonary tuberculosis by housing

Housing	Diseased	Not diseased	Total
Poor	30	70	100
Good	10	90	100

Controlling for a factor H while studying the influence of a factor E means to investigate the action of E separately on every level of H, that is in each subpopulation determined by one and the same value of H. The factor H is called a "confounder" for E if, by controlling for H, we obtain results for the action of E that are much different from those of the "uncontrolled" analysis of the influence of E where H is not involved.

We see that there is a somewhat arbitrary and not quantified element in the definition of a confounder since we have not made precise the meaning of "much" different. It is a matter of subjective appreciation in every concrete epidemiologic situation.

In our example housing (H) is certainly a confounder for education (E). It makes us believe in the influence of the factor education that in reality does not exist.

We can of course also control for education while studying the influence of housing. In the population consisting of persons with only primary education the risk of tuberculosis is $27/90 = 0.3$ among people in poor housing and $1/10 = 0.1$ in good housing, which gives a risk ratio of 3. In the population of subjects having received secondary education the corresponding risks are $3/10 = 0.3$ and $9/90 = 0.1$, which results again in the risk ratio 3. These risk ratios coincide with the risk ratio found above for the influence of housing without controlling for education. Thus, education is *not* a confounder for the action of the factor housing! Loosely speaking it is the factor housing and not the factor education that influences the prevalence of pulmonary tuberculosis.

Confounding is an almost universal phenomenon in epidemiologic studies. Very often, in order to really understand the influence of a factor, we have to control for others that may "confound" its action. The problem is important both in analytic studies where we want to learn about risk factors for a disease, and in experimental studies, especially in clinical trials where we study the effects of treatments. In the epidemiologic literature, many risk factors have been wrongly described as exerting an important influence because confounders were not sufficiently taken into account.

"Age" is one of the most frequently met confounders. In the following section we shall use the example of age in order to present a technique called "standardization" that amounts to constructing a summary of the process of controlling for a possible confounder. Standardization is treated in more detail in any book on "Population Science" (Demography), but its link with the idea of confounding in epidemiology is hardly ever mentioned. We shall restrict ourselves to the basic idea and deal only with a simplified situation.

Other confounders that appear frequently in epidemiologic practice are sex and various aspects of the socio-economic status.

21.2 Standardization

Vietnam is a "young" country and Germany an "old" one as defined by their age structure. We shall distinguish only two age groups: "young" will mean of age less than 45 and "old" is to mean at least 45. We can describe the age structure of the two countries around the year 2014 by the Table 21.4 of population numbers.

Table 21.4 Population around 2014

	Young	Old	Totals
Vietnam	v_y	v_z	v
Germany	g_y	g_z	g

According to the statistical services of the two countries, we have the following rounded figures in units "one million":

$$v_y = 61, \ v_z = 30, \ g_y = 40, \ g_z = 42, \ v = 91, \ g = 82$$

They show clearly that the proportion of old people was indeed much higher in Germany than in Vietnam; the first is $42/82 = 0.51$ but the second is only $30/91 = 0.33$.

The incidence of several diseases such as many types of cancer, cardio-vascular disorders, and diabetes mellitus increases with age. One can therefore suspect that when comparing risks in the two countries, the factor age acts as a confounder. Indeed even if the incidence rate (incidence density) were more or less the same for the two countries within each age group, the overall incidence rate for the whole country without controlling for age would certainly be greater in Germany.

To have something concrete in mind let us look at cancer of the colon. Its frequency is close to that of intestinal cancer in general since cancer of the small intestine is fairly rare. We represent it, by country and age group, in the Table 21.5.

It should be noted that neither Vietnam nor Germany has a central cancer registry; see Sect. 22.1. For Germany the Robert Koch-Institut publishes incidence figures by age groups on the basis of reports from regional institutions. For the year 2014 they are

$$b_y = 1,692 \ \text{and} \ b_z = 59,059, \ \text{hence} \ b = 60,751$$

Corresponding figures for Vietnam are apparently not available. For the purpose of illustrating the concept of standardization we may use fictitious figures. They are based on the idea, perhaps wrong, that the incidence *rates* in both age groups are more or less the same in Vietnam and in Germany. This gives us

$$a_y = 2,600 \ \text{and} \ a_z = 42,000, \ \text{hence} \ a = 44,600$$

We first calculate and compare the "risks" as expressed by the incidence rates of colon cancer in the two countries. In Vietnam it is $a/v = 0.000490$ and in Germany we have $b/g = 0.000741$. This difference represents the influence of the factor "country" without controlling for age. At first sight, the lower incidence rate in Vietnam could be due to many reasons: a healthier diet, more physical work, genetic disposition, incomplete reporting etc.

Table 21.5 Incidence of colon cancer in 2014

	Young	Old	Totals
Vietnam	a_y	a_z	a
Germany	b_y	b_z	b

However, let us control for age. This means comparing risks separately for every age group. For young people we get an incidence rate in Vietnam equal to $a_y/v_y = 0.000043$ and in Germany $b_y/g_y = 0.000042$. Among old people we have in Vietnam $a_z/v_z = 0.001400$ and in Germany $b_z/g_z = 0.001406$.

We now ask the following question. What would be the incidence rate of colon cancer in Germany if:

- Germany had the same age structure as Vietnam;
- In each age group the incidence rate in Germany would still be what it actually is?

In that case, Germany would have, in millions,

$$g_y^* = \frac{v_y}{v} g = 55 \text{ young and } g_z^* = \frac{v_z}{v} g = 27 \text{ old inhabitants;}$$

the reader may compare these numbers with the "real" numbers $g_y = 40$ and $g_z = 42$. Therefore, if Germany had the same age structure as Vietnam but still the incidence rates that it actually has, in 2014 there would have occurred,

$$b_y^* = \frac{b_y}{g_y} g_y^* = 2,326.5$$

cases among young people and

$$b_z^* = \frac{b_z}{g_z} g_z^* = 37,966.5$$

cases among old people, that is, $b^* = b_y^* + b_z^* = 40,293$ cases altogether, hence an incidence rate in Germany of $b^*/g = 0.000491$.

This number is called the incidence rate of colon cancer in Germany after "standardizing" by the age structure of Vietnam; the term "adjusting" is also being used. It is lower than the actual incidence rate 0.000741.

The actual, "non-standardized" incidence rate of colon cancer in Germany is designated as the "crude" incidence rate.

Standardizing an incidence rate in a human population G by the age structure of another human population V means calculating it again with the same incidence rates in every age group of G as before but assuming now that G had the age structure of V.

Instead of incidences, we can of course standardize prevalences, mortalities etc., and "age" can be replaced by other variables.

Often, one compares the disease situation in two countries with different age structures by using the age structure of a third country or region as the standard, for example that of the whole world. The latter is provided for this purpose by WHO or the United Nations (www.un.org/popin/data.html).

21.3 Practical Work

Using as a standard the age structure of the whole world with the three age groups
0–14, 15–64, 65–..., standardize the mortality per 100,000 inhabitants around the
year 2014 by cardio-vascular causes of the two countries Laos and Vietnam.
Compare the two and comment. Hint: For the mortality by cardio-vascular causes,
see Sect. 22.1.

Lesson 22
Epidemiology of Cancer

Cancer has become one of the main health burdens in Vietnam. Understanding its risk factors and applying this knowledge to primary and secondary prevention is vital.

22.1 Descriptive Epidemiology

Cancer registries are the main sources of indicators on incidence and mortality and, to some extent, on prevalence of the various forms of cancer.

They exist in many countries. The oldest one started operating in Denmark in 1943. The Vietnamese Cancer Registry is being built up gradually from regional registries that now function in Hanoi and Ho Chi Minh-City and in many municipal or provincial hospitals. Before the existence of cancer registries Ministries of Health relied on reported data from hospitals. Moreover, in some countries and for highly lethal forms of cancer, *mortality* indicators are being used to estimate incidences, too. Indeed, if almost every diseased subject eventually dies of the disease and if the situation remains more or less stable in time, the number of deaths in later years will be close to the number of new cases that appear earlier in a year.

Some cancer registries are exclusively based on routine reports from hospitals to the site of the registry; this is called "passive case finding". Other registries employ "active case finding". Thereby, staff of the registry will regularly visit all hospitals and clinics where cases of cancer are likely to be diagnosed and will collect the required information.

Due to these various sources of information and in spite of many gaps and errors, estimates of cancer incidences and mortalities are in general more reliable than those of other chronic diseases. They are centralized, aggregated, evaluated and published by the "International Agency for Research on Cancer" (IARC) in Lyon, France (www.iarc.fr/) and the "International Association of Cancer Registries (IACR)" in a series of books "Cancer Incidence in Five Continents", which come out about every 5 years. The last volume, No XI, covered the period 2008–2012. It presents only partial data about Vietnam. We therefore reproduce here an older

© Springer Nature Switzerland AG 2019
K. Krickeberg et al., *Epidemiology*, Statistics for Biology and Health,
https://doi.org/10.1007/978-3-030-16368-6_22

Table 22.1 Reported cancer incidence and mortality in 2002

	Incidence 2002				Mortality 2002			
	World		Vietnam		World		Vietnam	
Site	Male	Female	Male	Female	Male	Female	Male	Female
Lung	965,241	386,891	8089	3026	848,132	330,786	7480	2858
Colon, rectum	550,465	472,687	3428	2601	278,446	250,532	2220	1664
Stomach	603,419	330,518	6104	3159	446,052	254,297	5190	2661
Liver	442,119	184,043	6933	1827	416,882	181,439	6515	1720
Prostate	679,023		756		221,002		475	
Breast		1,151,298		5268		410,712		2284
Cervix		493,243		6224		273,505		3334
Ovaries		204,499		1446		124,860		810
All types	5,801,839	5,060,657	41,665	33,485	3,795,991	2,927,896	33,318	21,324

and more complete table about the situation in 2002, which may not be overly reliable, though. It gives incidences and mortalities by sex in the year 2002 in the whole world and in Vietnam for some of the most important sites of cancer (Table 22.1).

The worldwide incidence of all types of cancer in 2002 for both sexes together was near 11 million and mortality was near seven million. In Vietnam the corresponding numbers were about 90,000 and 55,000. The true incidences and mortalities were no doubt still higher.

The cancer mortality of over 55,000 in Vietnam in 2002 may for example be compared with the mortality in Vietnam by tuberculosis in 2007 as shown in table in Sect. 7.1, namely about 20,000. Thus cancer is certainly one of the main health burdens worldwide and in Vietnam.

Trends, that is, the evolution in time of cancer incidence and mortality depend not only on the type of cancer but also on the underlying target population. Regarding long-term trends in developing countries, information on a more distant past is scarce but there is certainly a strong general increase of incidence and mortality. This may be due in part to the demographic transition sketched in Sect. 1.2 since cancer is largely a disease of the elderly. However, it seems to be clear that the action of new risk factors also plays an important role; see Sect. 22.3, below.

The most prominent trends in recent times are the following:

- A decrease of the incidence of *stomach cancer* almost everywhere.
- For *lung cancer*: Stable state or decrease among men in developed countries; increase among men in developing countries and among women in both developing and developed countries.

The "survival time" after diagnosis is another aspect of the burden imposed on health in a given population by a given type of cancer. We shall not enter into details here because they are treated in clinical courses. Let us only remark that a common epidemiologic indicator determined by the survival time is the "5 year relative survival", that is the proportion of patients who are still alive 5 years after the diagnosis of their cancer. It depends not only on the type of cancer itself but also on diagnostic procedures, in particular existing screening programmes, and on the availability of treatments. Hence it is changing in time and there are important differences between countries. Here are some recent indicative values for Europe by site of the cancer: lung 5%; colon 43%; cervix 62%; breast 66%.

22.2 History and Attempts at Causal Analysis

The Latin word "cancer" denotes originally the animal but already the Roman physician Aulus Cornelius Celsus ($\approx$25 BC – $\approx$50 AC) whom we have already met in Sect. 4.1 and even the Roman poet Publius Ovidius Naso (43 BC – $\approx$17 AC) used it also in the sense of a tumour in humans. In this they followed Hippocrates ($\approx$460 – $\approx$375 BC) who employed the Greek name "karkinos" of the animal; this has given rise to the term "carcinoma", which nowadays means a malignant tumour that starts from epithelial tissue.

The history of cancer is indeed very old. Bone tumours have been identified in fossils and Egyptian human mummies. The oldest written description of cases of cancer, in fact breast cancer, was found on Egyptian papyri from around 1600 BC. Chinese drawings of tumours appear in the eleventh century BC and Chinese medical writings before 200 BC contain detailed descriptions of tumours and even putative causes. The nosology of cancer became more precise in the eighteenth century when autopsies could be performed. In the nineteenth century, the methods of cellular pathology developed by Rudolf Virchow (1821–1902) and the use of the microscope for examining tissue allowed better classification and diagnosis. They were essential for improving surgical treatment that had already been inaugurated by the Scottish surgeon John Hunter (1728–1793).

In this book we are interested in risk factors and prevention. We shall not dwell upon the many aetiological theories that have been advanced over the centuries, starting again with Hippocrates, but rather recall some concrete observations.

In the year 1713 the Italian physician Bernardino Ramazzini noticed that nuns had almost never cervical cancer but that the incidence of breast cancer among them was much higher than in the rest of the population. He conjectured that this was due to celibacy.

Sixty-two years later, the surgeon Percival Pott phrased his comparative observations in quantitative terms. He reported that scrotal cancer was very frequent among London chimney sweeps and that their mortality due to this disease was more than 200 times higher than that of other workers. In modern terms this was a rudimentary cohort study as described in Sect. 17.1 and the corresponding estimated risk ratio of death was over 200. His study also had a rapid application to primary prevention, namely the "Chimney Sweeper's Act" of 1788.

The risk factor "nicotine consumption" had a particularly heavy impact on both human health and on the evolution of the field of epidemiology. Warnings against the dangers of snuffing or smoking tobacco appeared frequently from the early seventeenth century on, for example in an Arabian text found in Timbuktu. In 1761 the physician, pharmacist, botanist and journalist John Hill published in London a pamphlet "Cautions against the Immoderate Use of Snuff", which concerned already some outcomes "cancer". Starting in the late nineteenth century a rapid increase of the incidence of lung cancer was noticed; before it had been a rare disease. In 1939 the German physician F. H. Müller published a paper on a link between smoking and lung cancer. An institute for research into the hazards of tobacco was founded in 1941 in the German university town of Jena. In 1943 it conducted the first modern study that showed this link very clearly. It was still a fairly simple case–control study but after that the British epidemiologists Richard Doll and Austin Bradford Hill confirmed the link beyond any doubt in two famous investigations: another case–control study, published in 1950, and the cohort study already described in Sect. 17.1 where they followed up smoking and non-smoking doctors from 1951 to 1964, and then extended their observations.

Let us still mention three examples from the recent history that will lead us to the present time to be taken up in the following section. They all concern forms of cancer of fairly high incidence.

The first one is colorectal cancer or colon cancer for short. Its interest for the epidemiologist resides in the profusion of potential risk factors that have been incriminated and investigated. The influence of smoking, alcohol, physical inactivity and polyps in the colon seems to be confirmed but in spite of very many studies the role of various diets still remains controversial.

On the contrary, for stomach cancer, a single prevailing pathogen has emerged, namely infection by the bacterium *Helicobacter pylori*. Before, many other theories, not founded on epidemiologic evidence, had been forwarded; they motivated useless or harmful therapies.

Our third example is liver cancer caused by HBV; see Lesson 9. Its peculiarity is the long asymptomatic stage after the infection that finally leads to liver diseases including cancer.

In the first half of the twentieth century the interest in the aetiology of cancer and causal analysis began to reach beyond the imaginative but unfounded theories of the past. The puzzling thing was the large variety of carcinogens. There were many chemical agents. Their study started in 1915 when a Japanese scientist induced cancer on rabbit skin by applying coal tar, thus complementing Percival Pott's results. There were also viruses. In 1911 Peyton Rous in New York attributed sarcoma in chickens to what later became known as the *Rous sarcoma virus*. The main evidence was, as Rous said in his Nobel Lecture in 1966, that there were "…malignant chicken sarcoma which could be propagated by transplanting its cells, these multiplying in their new hosts and forming new tumours of the same sort". Soon, radiations of all kind including light were shown to cause cancer. Genetic factors were found and hormonal disorders investigated that might explain Ramazzini's observations. Then the common final stage of the causal pathways along which these factors act was discovered:

Cancer is due to damaged and not repaired DNA in human cells, and the damage may be done directly or indirectly by any of many risk factors.

22.3 Specific Risk Factors

When trying to investigate suspected risk factors in a rigorous way we are in the area of observational studies. Practically every type of study has been used. Case–control studies have been playing a prominent role because the risks involved are usually small with the exception of those due to the factor "smoking". Several cohort studies like the one mentioned above by Doll and Hill were done, too. There were also "ecological studies" to evaluate the results of environmental exposure defined for an entire community; see Sect. 24.1.

In all of these studies, many possible confounding factors exist. However, in general the effects to be described below persist even after controlling for the more or less obvious confounders.

In the two preceding sections, we have mainly proceeded by *outcomes*. Let us now, in a more modern approach, arrange the material by *risk factors*.

We start with the *predisposition* to cancer of a subject, that is, existing genetic factors. Informal observations over the centuries have led to the belief that women in families where several cases of breast cancer have occurred are themselves more susceptible to breast cancer. Similar observations have been made for cancer of the colon and prostate cancer. Modern methods of genetic epidemiology to be sketched in Sect. 26.3 have confirmed this belief. In the beginning the old observations were made precise by proving that a so-called "familial aggregation" exists for these three types of cancer and for lung cancer. Then, many genes were identified whose inherited mutations increase the risk of some types of cancer considerably. In addition to those kinds of cancer already mentioned, this holds for skin cancer and sarcoma, too. Some estimates assert that on the whole inherited risk factors contribute about 10–15% of cancer incidence.

Next, we take up the discussion of the most terrible carcinogenic risk factor, *tobacco smoking*.

Tobacco smoking is by far the main single risk factor for cancer, both by the many types of cancer caused by it and by the high risks involved.

Here is a list of recognized sites of cancers that may be caused by smoking: bladder, cervix, kidney, larynx, liver, lung, nasal cavity, oesophagus, oral cavity, pancreas, pharynx and stomach; myeloid leukaemia can also be due to smoking.

When speaking about risk ratios we must of course make precise the concept of smoking. In many studies it is interpreted in the sense of "having ever smoked". This is reasonable because smoking is very habit forming. Most people who start smoking continue to do it. The reduction of the risk among those few who succeed in giving up smoking has also been investigated but we shall not discuss it here. The results of the many studies done vary a lot but in 2008 a meta-analysis (see Lesson 28) was published that gave the following estimations for the risk ratio r and the corresponding attributable fraction η among smokers for the incidence of the three types of highest risk: lung $r = 9$, $\eta = 89\%$; larynx $r = 7$, $\eta = 86\%$; the same for pharynx. More refined studies take into account the quantity of tobacco consumed by asking for example: "How many cigarettes do you habitually smoke per day?"

The total number of cases of cancer caused by smoking has also been investi-gated many times. Unlike the attributable fraction among smokers, it depends on how many people are smoking. A very conservative estimate from 1994 was that 15% of all cancers worldwide, that is about 1.5 million new cases per year, were due to smoking, in fact 16% in developed and 10% in developing countries It was 25% among men and 4% among women. As said before the situation is changing due to changing smoking habits.

Passive smoking, that is inhaling the smoke from other people who are smoking, is difficult to evaluate but several studies seem to indicate that it also exerts an essential influence on lung cancer.

Alcohol drinking increases the risk of cancer of the larynx, oesophagus, oral cav-ity, pharynx and probably others. This effect depends much on the quantity of alco-hol consumed habitually but apparently little on the type of drink, for example whether beer or hard liquor. We shall therefore not quote specific risk ratios and only mention that according to a recent estimate, 3.6% of all cases of cancer world-wide are due to alcohol.

Nutritional factors, also called *dietary factors*, have attracted the attention for a long time already. They present particularly difficult problems, though. An exposure by tobacco smoking or alcohol drinking is relatively easy to measure, even retrospectively, because people remember it more or less. By contrast, gen-eral nutritional exposures are hard to define and often impossible to measure ret-rospectively; people are often not sure about their dietary habits in the past. These habits may also vary during the life of a person. For some more comments see Sect. 25.2. Therefore, case–control studies are rarely adapted to investigate the influence of a dietary factor on such and such cancer and one has to revert to long-lasting cohort studies. Moreover, a normal diet contains many components and it is usually difficult to separate their influence from each other. As a result, the action of nutritional factors on cancer remains largely uncertain and often contro-versial. We shall just mention some facts that seem to be established well but shall not give quantitative indications on risk ratios.

In 1997 a survey of results about the influence of about 30 nutritional compo-nents on the risks of 14 types of cancers was published. The nutritional compo-nents included the traditional ones such as vegetables, fruit, sugar, fat, meat, eggs, fish, milk, coffee, black and green tea, but also more modern categories like starch, fibres, saturated fat, animal protein and finally micronutrients, that is vitamins, minerals and trace elements. Four kinds of evidence were defined: convincing, probable, possible, and insufficient; however, for most components of food and types of cancer, no indication about evidence was given. The only convincing evi-dence concerned the influence of vegetables and fruit, which *decrease* the risk of cancer of the lung, the oesophagus and the oral cavity and pharynx; vegetables also have such an influence on cancer of the colon and rectum. Vegetables and fruit probably decrease as well the risk of cancer of the bladder, breast and pancreas. There are probable effects in the sense of an *increase* of the risk by meat on cancer of the colon and rectum, and by coffee on cancer of the stomach. This paucity of results reflects the difficulties of epidemiologic studies sketched above. On the borderline of nutritional factors we have aflotoxins produced by fungi of the genus *aspergillus* that grow on organic waste, rotten food, peanuts etc.; they may raise the risk of liver cancer.

Since the middle of the 1990s a very large cohort study involving about 520,000 persons in 10 European countries (European Prospective Investigation into Cancer and Nutrition) is being conducted. Its preliminary results confirm some of the facts mentioned before but not all of them; this underlines again the difficulties inherent in the subject.

There has been much concern about carcinogenic effects of *additives* to food. Well over one thousand of them are being employed for conservation, colouring, changing the texture or stretching a product, or influencing its taste. Monosodium glutamate and saccharin are classical examples. Some are completely synthetic, others are obtained by modifying natural substances, e.g. so-called "natural" colours. Many were shown to induce various forms of cancer in animals but for the difficulties described above, rigorous epidemiologic studies in human populations are rare.

Overweight is a risk factor related to nutrition. It increases the risk of colon cancer, cancer of the breast, kidney, and endometrium. However quantitative estimates fluctuate a lot. For instance an estimate made in 2001 indicated that in Europe over 6% of all cases of cancer in women and over 3% of all cases in men are due to overweight. Around the year 2016 it was reported that in the USA 8% of all cases result from overweight whereas a study in England gave only about 5%.

Occupational risk factors are being treated in every course on "Occupational Health". Here we shall restrict ourselves to a few general remarks. These risk factors are mostly chemical agents or mixtures plus a few physical ones such as dust, radiation, heat and noise. In general, the exposure can be defined and measured much more precisely than that by nutritional factors. Hence many studies, even long cohort studies, exist. Among the well-established results let us mention those on asbestos particles in the air, which is essentially the only causal agent of cancer of the mesothelium of the pleura and other organs. Asbestos also leads to a higher risk of lung cancer.

Next, there are *environmental risk factors*. Many occupational risk factors are in fact environmental factors at the work place. Also, most environmental risk factors for the general population are the result of industrial production processes. Examples are waste gas and fumes from factories and traffic, radiation, and waste disposals. Hundreds of manufactured chemical products like pesticides, plastic material, and cosmetics and synthetic building material are suspected of being carcinogenic. There exist *natural* environmental factors, too, such as pollen and radon radiation.

The study of any environmental factors in the general population is difficult for the same reasons that hamper those on nutritional factors. The exposures are usually low and hard to measure. They accumulate and often fluctuate during the life of a subject.

On the whole it seems that in general populations the influence of environmental risk factors on cancer incidence is relatively small compared with that of other factors. The situation is different in special populations that are particularly exposed to a specific natural or man-made risk factor from the environment. For example drinking water containing arsenic in some regions of Taiwan, Bangladesh, Vietnam and the French Massif Central apparently raises the risk of cancer of the bladder, kidney, liver, lung and perhaps even of the skin. Exposure to dioxin from the Orange Agent in Vietnam has lead to higher risks of various forms of cancer. Radiation around Hiroshima and Nagasaki after the atomic bombs in 1945 and around Chernobyl and Fukushima after the accidents of their nuclear power plants in April 1986 and March 2011, respectively, influenced cancer incidence in various ways.

Medical activities, too, may create risk factors for cancer. Like occupational factors they can be studied fairly well because exposures are in general clearly defined and recorded. X-rays for diagnostic purposes imply relatively small risks when used carefully and obeying strict rules, whereas radiotherapy increases the risk in the organs treated. The effects of drug and hormone treatments have been investigated extensively, for example for contraceptives, growth hormones, cancer chemotherapy and immunosuppressive drugs. We shall not enter into the fairly complicated details.

Infectious microorganisms have already appeared in the preceding section. Let us enumerate the main ones according to current knowledge. Among viruses, HBV can cause liver cancer (Lesson 9) and HIV can induce Kaposi's sarcoma and non-Hodgkin's lymphoma (Lesson 10). The majority of cases of cancer of the cervix are due to the human papillomavirus (HPV). The Epstein-Barr virus causes Burkitt's lymphoma and Hodgkin's disease. More than half of all cases of stomach cancer are the result of the action of the bacterium *H. pylori*. Some parasites also act on cancer of the bladder and of the liver. This enumeration is certainly not final.

Taken together, infectious agents play an important role in carcinogenesis, both in developed countries and even more in developing ones. Preliminary global estimates point to around 16% of all cancers as being due to infections.

Socio-economic risk factors have also been studied. Questions of the type "are poorer people more likely to develop stomach cancer" have some interest. However, it is more revealing to study the influence of social factors not on cancer but on known carcinogenic risk factors. We may for example ask: how do socio-economic determinants influence smoking habits, alcohol consumption, diet, overweight and occupational and environmental carcinogenic risk factors? This means that we investigate an entire "pathway", also called "causal chain", from socio-economic factors to cancer through intermediate steps. In the following lesson on cardiovascular diseases we shall treat the corresponding problem more in detail.

As almost everywhere in this book, we have restricted ourselves to looking at actions of a *single* factor; see the Foreword, Sect. 15.2 and Lesson 28. However, cancer epidemiology is a field where as a rule several factors act together. For example, genetic susceptibility interacts with many other risk factors. We cannot make this precise here.

22.4   Conclusions Regarding Primary and Secondary Prevention

Recall from Sect. 2.3 that "primary prevention" means reducing the level of harmful factors or eliminating them completely in order to lower the incidence of the disease in question. When going through the various categories of risk factors described in the preceding section, we see that in principle, with the exception of genetic factors and a few naturally occurring environmental ones, all of them are man-made and can be influenced by man. To which extent it is really being done depends on political decisions and socio-economic conditions.

Lowering the level of the factor "tobacco smoking" can be achieved by good health education and by legislative measures such as prohibiting to smoke in all public places, restricting the sale of cigarettes to a few special shops, eliminating all publicity for cigarettes and taxing cigarettes heavily while also suppressing the black market and smuggling. Although these measures meet everywhere in the world with strong resistance from the tobacco industry, they have had partial success in most developed countries. In Vietnam the Government Resolution No. 12/2000/NQ-CP of the 14 August 2000 on "National Tobacco Control Policy 2000–2010" outlined the strategy to follow. In 2012 and 2013 decrees to implement this resolution were issued but their impact until now is not easy to evaluate.

Reducing the carcinogenic factor "tobacco smoking" is one of the most efficient measures of primary prevention that can be taken at the present time.

Similar comments apply to the drinking of alcohol. The problem may be less severe, though, because alcohol at low doses is not as much habit forming as nicotine and perhaps also less harmful.

For nutritional and environmental factors, we refer to Lesson 25 and for occupational ones to any course on "Occupational Health".

For infectious agents, the method of choice is to control the spread of the infection in the target population. This was discussed in Lesson 9 for hepatitis B and in Lesson 10 for HIV/AIDS. In the case of infections by *H. pylori* early treatment by antibiotics has been very successful.

For cervical cancer there has recently been strong pressure to apply immunization against an infection by the human papillomavirus (HPV) to all young women but the efficacy and cost-effectiveness of this measure is as yet doubtful. The long-range efficiency of the immunization is still not known and frequent costly re-immunization may be necessary. It is quite possible that investing in good health education and in the classical screening programme described below will turn out to be more useful. There is also the danger that vaccinated young women will feel "protected", engage in riskier sexual behaviour and neglect their screening.

"Secondary prevention" is tantamount to screening for early detection and early intervention. Cancer evolves in general slowly and in several stages. The first stages need not yet be neoplastic and malignant. Efficient treatments in early stages exist for many types of cancer. Screening appears therefore especially promising when methods for early detection can be found.

However, before implementing or continuing a screening programme several elements need to be taken into account. Let us return to the general discussion in Sect. 19.3 and extend it in the concrete case of cancer. Cost and side effects, for example by X-rays, must be considered. There is also the danger that pre-cancerous lesions are discovered and treated, for example by surgery, that would not have developed into a full cancer before the death of the patient from other reasons, thus causing unnecessary disability.

A screening programme ought to be *evaluated* with respect to several criteria. The ideal evaluation is an experimental cohort study with the outcome "mortality" or "survival time". One cohort will consist of people who are screened and the other cohort includes those who are not. Early studies of this kind were done for breast cancer screening. They are not always feasible, though, partly for ethical reasons (Sect. 27.5) because they imply that people in one group are deprived of early diagnoses, and partly because they would have to last very long. Moreover, they provide information on the efficacy of the programme under the conditions of the study but in practice the selection of persons to seek a screening examination works very differently. There is the so-called "self-selection" effect, which means that healthier subjects and subjects of higher educational and social standing will participate in screening more frequently than others. This might have some bearing on the "effectiveness" of the programme in practice. Case-control studies and comparative intervention trials have also being conducted.

In the light of these arguments, let us look at the main screening programmes that have been organized or debated in many countries for the following types of cancer: breast, cervical, colorectal, lung, prostate and skin.

Screening for *breast cancer* relies mainly on mammography but also on physical inspection by palpation and, more recently, on sonography (ultrasound scan). It has been the subject of many evaluation studies including several large cohort studies. The first one, the so-called HIP (Health Insurance Plan)-trial in the USA, started in 1963 with over 30,000 women aged between 40 and 64 years in each group. It lasted 10 years and concluded that screening reduced mortality by breast cancer by about 30%. Later similar studies gave similar results. There seems to be agreement that screening by mammography in women older than 50 years is effective in the sense of a reduction of the mortality.

Screening for *cervical cancer* was put onto solid grounds already in 1943 by the book "Diagnosis of Uterine Cancer by the Vaginal Smear" by George Papanicolaou and Herbert Traut. It appears to be particularly suitable because there is a long period of years or even decades during which pre-cursor lesions can be detected and successfully treated. It is also relatively simple and free of side effects.

The older studies of the effectiveness of such a screening programme for cervical cancer are all community studies with historic controls; see Lesson 24. In the Nordic countries Denmark, Finland, Iceland, Norway and Sweden the mortality by cancer of the cervix after the implementation of the programme was compared with that before. The reduction of the mortality was between 30% (Denmark) and 73% (Iceland) with the exception of Norway (8%). Later case-control studies around 1980 in many developed countries yielded in general even higher reductions up to

80%. In Columbia, a reduction of 90% was found and in Thailand 28%. Nowadays one considers screening women over 25 years of age every 2 or 3 years to be the most reasonable approach.

For *colorectal cancer*, one of the two following screening methods is being recommended for individuals over 50 years of age up to 75 but not over 75. The first one is an annual examination of the faeces for occult blood. The second one consists of a visual inspection by a flexible coloscope (sigmoidoscopy). The first method suffers from a relatively low sensitivity and specificity (see Sect. 19.2). The second one is expensive. It is particularly useful in high-risk groups, for example among subjects that have suffered from polyps in the rectum or colon.

No screening method with sufficiently confirmed high effectiveness has yet been devised for *lung cancer*.

For *cancer of the prostate*, the traditional method of screening is digital, that is, by the finger of the physician in a rectal examination. Looking for the presence of the "prostate-specific antigen" (PSA) in the blood is the modern approach. The effectiveness of both is still being much debated, partly because of the danger of inappropriate early treatment mentioned in Sect. 19.3.

Some screening for *skin cancer* is for instance being done in Australia where people are often exposing themselves a lot to the sun and its ultraviolet light. It is also offered in several European countries by the general health insurance system.

22.5   Practical Work

1. Visit your provincial hospital and describe its system of cancer registration and cancer reporting.
2. Try to estimate the percentage of smokers in your vicinity. Both the target population and the method are left to your imagination.
3. Write a little report on visible educational measures in your commune or part of town aimed at reducing the habit of smoking.
4. Describe the screening programmes for cancer that exist in a district, starting with educational measures on the primary health care level in order to motivate people to participate.

Lesson 23
Epidemiology of Cardiovascular Diseases

Preventing cardiovascular diseases is now one of the main tasks of the Vietnamese health system. It rests on knowledge of their epidemiology.

23.1 Descriptive Epidemiology and Burden

It is not easy to present the essential features of the descriptive epidemiology of cardiovascular diseases succinctly and clearly. The exposition that follows will necessarily be rather cursory. There are two reasons for that. Firstly, several categories of these diseases exist whose epidemiology is quite different. Secondly, in many countries, in particular in Vietnam, the role of cardiovascular diseases is changing extremely fast.

There are indeed many categories of cardiovascular diseases such as cardiomyopathies, rheumatic heart disease and arrhythmia but we shall restrict ourselves to those of highest importance to Public Health at the present time:

The cardiovascular diseases that present the highest health burden are "coronary (ischaemic) heart diseases" and "stroke" (cerebrovascular events).

Coronary heart disease consists in reduced blood supply to the myocardium, which may lead to myocardial infarction or chronic heart failure. Stroke is the interruption of blood flow in the brain by thrombosis or haemorrhage.

In addition, there are two main "conditions" that we may regard alternately as risk factors, precursors or part of the disease:

The principal conditions leading to the outcomes above are "atherosclerosis" and "hypertension".

Atherosclerosis consists in hardening, loss of elasticity, thickening and reduced interior cross-section of arteries. It may lead to thrombosis.

Definitions of *hypertension* have been varying but at present there is fairly wide agreement, in particular in Vietnam, that it starts with a systolic blood pressure of over 140 mmHg or a diastolic blood pressure of over 90 mmHg, irrespective of age and sex. It may cause haemorrhage and thus lead to cerebrovascular events.

© Springer Nature Switzerland AG 2019
K. Krickeberg et al., *Epidemiology*, Statistics for Biology and Health,
https://doi.org/10.1007/978-3-030-16368-6_23

The two conditions are not independent of each other; for example loss of elasticity is connected with hypertension. Details of the complex clinical picture of the various aspects of cardiovascular diseases cannot be given here.

The second fact that prevents a simple epidemiologic description of cardiovascular diseases is the rapid change of their frequency. Figures concerning a given year may be far from those found 5 years earlier. This phenomenon is part of the "epidemiologic transition" described in Sect. 1.2. It consists of the shift in the burden of disease and in particular in mortality from the classical infectious diseases to noninfectious ailments, especially cardiovascular diseases that accompany demographic, social and economic change. It started in the middle of the twentieth century. For example, in the USA, cardiovascular diseases accounted for about 20% of all deaths in 1940 but already for 44% in 1948. At present, the latter percentage represents more or less the situation in the whole world, that is, almost half of all deaths are due to cardiovascular diseases. Mortality from coronary heart diseases is more or less of the same order of magnitude in all regions of the world whatever their state of development may be, and mortality from stroke is even higher in some developing countries than in developed ones.

A crucial question to be asked is whether this evolution results only from the "*demographic* transition" because cardiovascular diseases increase with age or whether there are other factors such as changing diets that contribute to it. Standardization (Sect. 21.2) of incidence, prevalence and mortality indicators by age is needed in order to answer this question. We shall come back to it in the following section.

The table in Sect. 1.2 provided a closer view of the relative weight of the main cardiovascular diseases. The mortality caused by them was compared to that from the other eight main causes. For the year 2016 the table gave the mortality as equal to 15 million worldwide by coronary heart diseases and stroke together; note that the total number of deaths from all causes was around 57 million. For comparison, the World Heart Federation had furnished for 2005 the figure of 17.5 million deaths worldwide from all cardiovascular diseases with about five million deaths by stroke.

Regarding Vietnam, in 2012 there were, according to the WHO, about 190 reported deaths by cardiovascular diseases per 100,000 inhabitants. However, when comparing mortalities in different countries, crude figures are not very illuminating and we ought to use indicators that are standardized by age; see Sect. 21.2. Let us just look at one example due to the statistical information system WHOSIS of WHO. In the year 2002, the age-standardized mortality from cardiovascular diseases per 100,000 inhabitants was 211 in Germany and 318 in Vietnam.

Many of these indicators are not very reliable, which also explains apparent inconsistencies in the figures presented by different sources. In particular, in Vietnam the system of collecting data and deriving indicators about cardiovascular diseases is still incomplete. In addition to indicators in the Health Statistics Yearbooks of the Ministry of Health that are based on reports from hospitals, there have been early surveys by the Vietnamese Association of Cardiologists and later ones supported by WHO. Partial information points to an important increase of the burden by cardiovascular diseases. For example, the percentage of people aged over

25 suffering from hypertension was 16% in the year 2000, 23% in 2002 (data from Hanoi only) and 25% in 2008. Between 1980 and 1990, 108 cases of acute myocardial infarction were admitted to the National Institute of Cardiology, but 82 cases in the much shorter period from 1991 to 1995.

Let us conclude the present section by a more systematic overview of the *methods* of the descriptive epidemiology of these diseases. As for all disease statistics a clear "case validation" is required in the first place. This amounts to putting every case into one of the categories of a given classification of diseases like the "International Classification of Diseases" (Sect. 1.2). To which extent it can always be done in practice depends on the state of the health system in which we are operating; there are great differences between countries. An example will be presented in the following section where we look at a link between diabetes and cardiovascular diseases.

Indicators on *mortality* by coronary heart disease or stroke are obtained routinely from the so-called "vital statistics" based on death certificates. For many countries they are fairly reliable.

For indicators on the *prevalence* of conditions such as atherosclerosis, hypertension or chronic heart failure, cross-sectional surveys are being employed and usually repeated periodically in order to investigate trends. Cohort studies provide information on *incidence* of coronary heart diseases and stroke. All of these studies serve at the same time to investigate the influence of risk factors; this is the subject of the next section.

23.2 Determinants and their Studies

We are confronted with a large variety of confirmed or suspected risk factors. Their influence on the target diseases and the manifold connections between them are the subject of much ongoing research and are far from being elucidated.

We have already observed that *age* is an important risk factor for cardiovascular diseases; their frequency generally increases with age. Hence higher life expectancy and the demographic transition contribute to higher overall incidence and prevalence in most countries. The main topic of contemporary epidemiologic studies is, however, the role of *other* factors. How do they act when we control for age?

The list of suspected or confirmed risk factors for cardiovascular diseases is indeed long. The history of their exploration has been shaped to a large extent by a few particularly prominent and revealing studies. We shall therefore structure the present section by *studies*, in contrast to what we did in the preceding Sect. 22.4 on cancer, which was structured by *risk factors*. To start with studies may also be a more lively and attractive approach than to go through the determinants one by one.

Over the centuries there have been many observations and more or less rigorous small studies on the aetiology and on risk factors for cardiovascular diseases.

One can trace them back to the early eighteenth century but it was only in the second half of the twentieth century that one began to investigate the epidemiology of cardiovascular diseases systematically. A famous observation published in 1957 compared men of Japanese descent who lived in Japan, Hawaii and California, respectively. Their mortality by coronary heart disease was low in Japan, intermediate in Hawaii and high in California. The opposite was true for mortality by stroke. It could thus be argued that the differences were due to the geographical factor but not to genetic differences between persons of Japanese and non-Japanese ancestry. The geographical factor, in turn, might act via environmental or life style differences.

The longest cohort study started in 1948 in the community of Framingham, Massachusetts, USA; it is still going on. At that time Framingham counted about 28,000 inhabitants. Over 5200 people in the age group 30–59 years who were free of any heart disease were recruited in the beginning by a sampling plan. The following main risk factors were registered for every subject in the study: cholesterol concentration in the blood, blood pressure, alcohol and tobacco consumption, weight and physical activities. Their levels defined the cohorts to be followed. Outcomes were measured every 2 years. In the year 1971 the study population was renewed by adding over 5100 children of the original subjects. In 2002 about 3500 grandchildren came in.

One of the first essential results appeared already in 1960, namely that *cigarette smoking* raises the risk of cardiovascular diseases. Shortly afterwards, the same kind of result could be established for the risk factors *hypertension* and *high cholesterol level*. The particular influence of hypertension on stroke was further elucidated a few years later. In 1977 the different action of low-density lipoprotein cholesterol (supposed to be "bad") and high-density lipoprotein cholesterol (supposed to be "good") was described. The beneficial effects of *physical activities* and the harmful effects of *overweight* had already become clear in 1970. The following interesting fact in the area of descriptive epidemiology appeared: while it had been known that men in general have a higher risk of cardiovascular diseases than women, this difference virtually disappears after menopause because the risk in women is then increasing.

Later on risk factors of a different kind were added to the "classical" ones listed before, in particular *psychosocial* factors and *genetic* ones. For example it turned out that hard-driving and competitive behaviour, impatience and hostility increase the risk of coronary heart diseases.

Three more large studies were conducted over a long time or are still going on. The first one was the Whitehall Study of British civil servants, which focussed on socio-economic factors and will be described in Sect. 26.2. It was a cohort study.

The second one was the Seven Countries Study in order to investigate factors which may underlie the differences in coronary heart diseases in European, Japanese and North American populations. It started in 1958 in Finland, Greece, Italy, Japan, The Netherlands, the USA and Yugoslavia. The study population consisted of nearly 13,000 men aged from 40 to 59 years. Sixteen cohorts were constructed and followed for up to 25 years. However, this was not a person-based cohort study as we have treated them in Lesson 17 but an ecological population-based study in the sense of Lesson 24, that is, the risk factors were defined and measured for the entire cohorts, not for their individual members. A minor person-based component was added later. The study dealt mainly with *dietary patterns* in addition to the geographical factor and smoking. In particular the role of the so-called "Mediterranean diet" was to be investigated, which is characterized by a low consumption of red meat and emphasis on bread, beans, nuts, vegetables, fruit, fish, olive oil and small quantities of wine. The outcome variables were incidence of, and mortality from, coronary heart diseases. Some of the main results are as follows: consumption of red meat is an important risk factor and so are the eating of much saturated fat, elevated serum cholesterol levels and smoking. High fish consumption, especially of "fatty" fish such as herring and mackerel, lowers the risk of dying from coronary heart disease. Regarding the influence of the *geographical factor*, the age-adjusted mortality rate from coronary heart diseases over a period of 25 years was for example 5% in the Greek island of Crete and in a community in Japan but 29% in Eastern Finland.

The third study to be mentioned is the MONICA Project (MONItoring Trends and Determinants in CArdiovascular Disease) of WHO. Its main purpose was to investigate *trends*, that is changes in time, of risk factors, of the outcomes "coronary heart disease" and "stroke" and of the *connection* between trends in risk factors and trends in outcomes. They were studied in populations; in other words this study, too, was population-based. It used two types of study designs in parallel. One of them consisted in repeated cross-sectional sample surveys. The other one exploited surveillance mechanisms in hospitals. The target population was composed of 38 well-defined subpopulations of together roughly ten million people aged 35–64 years in 21 countries. The samples had a size of about 1000–3000 subjects. After an initial survey in the years 1979–1989 there was a main and final survey starting in the mid-1980s with a follow-up of 10 years. Thus MONICA does not cover the most recent trends.

In agreement with the idea of an epidemiologic transition, trends are not the same, and in fact largely opposite, in developed and developing countries. The states of the former Soviet Union and some East European countries occupy a particular place. They suffer from especially high incidence of, and mortality from, coronary heart disease; opinions about the role of the various risk factors remain controversial. Results of the MONICA Project in most developed countries show a recent decrease in factors such as hypertension, smoking and cholesterol levels together with a decrease in mortality from coronary heart diseases while obesity is still increasing. The MONICA Project in China did not establish clear-cut trends because of very large variation between different regions.

Summarizing the main findings by the MONICA Project we may say that the prominent known determinants like smoking, high total cholesterol, overweight and hypertension are responsible for the bulk of the incidence of, and mortality by, coronary heart disease. Moreover, changes in coronary heart events correspond to changes of these determinants on the population level.

As already remarked in the beginning of Sect. 23.1, the epidemiology of cardiovascular diseases is progressing rapidly. Many studies were completed or are going on in addition to those that we have just described. Thus, the overall picture is complex. Sometimes a result of a study is not confirmed or even contradicted by another one, and the role of various determinants is being fiercely debated. Still, the "classical" factors listed above still play a major role.

Let us also quote recent interesting results about connections between cardiovascular diseases and diabetes of type 2. Firstly, both share many risk factors such as obesity, wrong diets and hypertension. Secondly, more than 70% of type 2 diabetes patients die of cardiovascular diseases. This causes a problem of *case validation*: what was the primary cause of death of these people?

Newer investigations concern above all questions of *pathways* and *causation* analogously to what we had met in the epidemiology of cancer. For example, as pointed out in the preceding section, the "conditions" atherosclerosis and hypertension are risk factors for coronary heart disease or stroke. At the same time they may be outcomes of the action of "primary" determinants such as smoking. A high cholesterol level and, more precisely, the so-called "metabolic syndrome" can also be looked upon as an intermediate step in a pathway.

The principal categories of "primary" risk factors for cardiovascular diseases at the "root" of pathways are *age, sex, ethnicity, smoking, dietary imbalance, physical inactivity* **and** *psychosocial* **and** *socio-economic* **factors.**

Let us add some remarks on these; we can of course not enter into details. We have already quoted an early observation to the effect that ethnicity may play a minor role compared with factors of life-style and environment. This has been confirmed by later studies and holds for other genetic factors, too.

Regarding nutrition, let us summarize the essential:

The main harmful components of an imbalanced diet are salt, red meat, saturated fats and excessive energy intake.

The role of psychosocial and socio-economic factors was examined relatively late. The Whitehall studies focussed in the beginning on general mortality, and the outcome "coronary heart disease" appeared only in its second part. The Framingham study, too, included social factors very late. They were investigated extensively by the more recent MONICA-Project. In the end, the influence of social factors was established in many forms. For example, it turned out that in the USA well-educated people have lower risks of dying from coronary heart disease than less educated ones. The question of the pathway poses itself again: do well-educated Americans smoke less, eat more reasonably and are more active physically than the less educated, which in turn influences their mortality by coronary heart diseases? Interestingly enough, even after controlling for those factors as possible confounders, educated persons are still at an advantage.

The biophysical and biochemical mechanisms at work in the various steps of a pathway are far from having been elucidated, and are not the subject of the present book on epidemiology.

23.3 Prevention and Public Health Measures

Several specialized organizations devoted to cardiovascular diseases have issued recommendations and guidelines for primary or secondary prevention of cardiovascular events and deaths. Primary prevention means acting on the risk factors sketched above. Thus, the relevant recommendations concern in the first place smoking, wrong diets, lack of physical activities and overweight but also monitoring of blood pressure and cholesterol concentrations. Secondary prevention amounts to screening in suspected high-risk populations; this is still being neglected almost everywhere. Instead, a follow-up and treatment of individuals who have already suffered a non-fatal coronary heart attack or stroke is being practised more widely (tertiary prevention).

Most of these recommendations stem from organizations in Europe and the USA. The situation in Vietnam is different. Smoking was on the rise until a few years ago but now seems to decline slowly. Diets are changing rapidly, mainly to the worse; we shall come back to this in Sect. 25.2. Overweight makes its appearance. Hence specific Vietnamese recommendations need to be developed and widely spread by modern methods of health education. Many of the remarks made in Sect. 22.4 apply here as well; the problem is mainly political.

There have also been many intervention programmes on a community level and community trials in order to evaluate them. We cannot approach this subject here; for the general idea see Lesson 24.

23.4 Practical Work

1. Health education campaigns can be organized specifically for a given risk factor, for example smoking, or be combined for several risk factors such as smoking and wrong diet. Likewise, it can be done for a specific type of outcomes, for example cancer, or combined for several outcomes such as cancer and cardiovascular diseases. Give arguments for and against campaigns which are

   – conducted jointly for smoking and wrong diet;
   – conducted jointly for cancer and cardiovascular diseases.

2. Inform yourself about the activities of the Vietnamese Association of Cardiologists and describe its activities in the domain of epidemiology and prevention.
3. Study preventive activities in your Commune Health Station and District Hospital.

Lesson 24
Community Studies

In a community study, also called ecological study, both the exposure and the outcome concern communities as a whole, not single persons.

24.1 The Concept of a Community Study

Up to now we have almost exclusively dealt with "person-based" studies. By this we mean that both the variable "risk factor"and the variable "health outcome"are defined for individual persons, who are human beings. Typical factors are age, nicotine consumption, housing standard, a diagnosis and a medical treatment received, defined for each person in the target population. Likewise, the outcome, which may for example be the appearance of lung cancer or the cure from malaria, concerns individuals. Studying the influence of a factor means comparing the frequency of the outcome in subgroups determined by different levels of the factor; see Sect. 15.1.

However, there are factors and outcomes that do not fit into this mould. Let us look at five examples. All of them concern the province of Thai Binh.

First, suppose the Health Department of the province asks all of its Commune Health Stations to launch a special educational campaign for the prevention of AIDS, in addition to the usual information on television and in newspapers. It may consist of messages disseminated by posters, written information distributed to households, or home visits by health workers. An outcome may be the yearly incidence of AIDS in the communes during the subsequent next 5 years.

A second example might be a similar campaign to promote healthy nutrition in order to reduce the incidence of certain forms of cancer or cardiovascular diseases. Here, information provided in schools can play an important role, too.

As a third example let us mention a campaign in order to lower the number and severity of traffic accidents; see Sect. 3.1.

A fourth example is education in the context of the programme CDD; see Sect. 6.4. There, mothers need to be made aware that the main danger in a case of diarrhoea is dehydration, that they should not deprive the young patients of drinks, and

© Springer Nature Switzerland AG 2019
K. Krickeberg et al., *Epidemiology*, Statistics for Biology and Health,
https://doi.org/10.1007/978-3-030-16368-6_24

that a very simple and cheap method of rehydration exists, which is available at their Commune Health Station or hospital.

As a fifth example, education for better hygiene is a classical but still very actual theme (Sects. 2.1 and 2.3).

In these examples the value of a certain determinant, namely an "educational campaign" in a commune, and the outcome, for example an incidence in it, concern the commune as a whole, not an individual person. These variables are defined on the "set", or "collection", of all communes of the province of Thai Binh, which is now our "target set".

In a general setting we deal with a target set whose elements are communities, that is, populations. Studies in order to investigate the influence of any factors defined on such a target set are then called "community studies". Another term is "ecological study", which is derived from the Greek word "*oicos*" for house. Sometimes the expression "cross-population study" is being used but we shall avoid it.

In a community study both the risk factor and the health outcome are defined for entire communities, that is, for groups or populations of people, not for individual persons.

Therefore, such studies are called "community-based" or "population-based".

In the five examples above each input variable has the form of an *intervention* in certain communities, which are communes in the sense of administration. We are dealing here with *experimental* community studies because the input variable, that is the factor "intervention", is being created by the investigator; see Sect. 18.1. Studies of this kind are being called "intervention studies" or "intervention trials". They will be treated further in the following section.

There also exist *observational*, or *analytic*, community-based studies. Here, the factor to be studied exists independently of any intervention of the health system. It may be the geographical location of the community at hand, or the climate, the presence of stagnant water nearby, air or water pollution, polluting industry in the vicinity, or certain socio-economic factors which concern the community as a whole such as a good level of public schooling or the existence and type of social networks. The Seven Countries Study of cardiovascular diseases described in Sect. 23.2 is an excellent example. For more examples, see Sects. 25.3 and 26.2.

The factors that we have listed as examples are defined *directly* for entire communities and have no meaning for individual persons. Factors of this kind play an important role in modern social epidemiology; see Sect. 26.2. However, many risk factors which concern entire communities are derived from factors defined originally for individual people or households. They usually have the form of an *average* over the community in question. Typical examples are the average weight of people in a given age group of a commune, the average income of the households there, the average size of houses in a part of a city, and the percentage of people in a district having received secondary education. Most risk factors investigated in older ecological studies are of this type. Regarding outcome variables they are almost always obtained by averaging person-based outcomes. They are indeed defined as incidences, prevalences, mortalities, life expectancies and the like as in the examples sketched above.

When should we organize a community study? Often it just appears natural because it fits exactly the problem we are facing. This was the case in our five examples above. For other problems a person-based study may be impossible for technical reasons. This happens mainly in register-based studies. In a person-based study we do indeed need, for every individual person, *both* the value of the risk factor *and* the one of the outcome variable. The available registers rarely provide it. Often, however, there exists, for certain communities, information in some statistical office about indicators connected with risk factors and in another office we can find indicators about outcomes such as incidences in the same communities. This allows a community-based study, usually of the retrospective cohort type. They are frequent in environmental and social epidemiology. Examples will be given in Lesson 26, in particular at the end of Sect. 26.2.

The result of a community study is sometimes considered a first clue about a possible action of person-based factors, too. For example, if we find that countries with higher cigarette consumption per adult inhabitant also have a higher mortality by lung cancer, we should suspect that smoking raises the risk of dying from lung cancer for individual persons as well.

This type of reasoning may lead to wrong conclusions, though, which we call "ecological fallacies".

An ecological fallacy is a wrong conclusion drawn from a community study about the influence of a risk factor on a health outcome defined for individual subjects.

It is indeed intuitively obvious that a single indicator such as an average for an entire community conveys less information than the underlying data about *every* member of the community together.

Ecological fallacies have been frequent in the history of epidemiology. Let us look at a fictitious example. Suppose that in a certain country both the average cigarette consumption and mortality from lung cancer are high. It is well conceivable that the elevated consumption of cigarettes stems from a few smokers who smoke enormously much but never attract lung cancer whereas the high mortality from lung cancer concerns non-smokers and is due to other causes. Then we cannot conclude that smoking is a "strong" risk factor for lung cancer. Arguments of this kind were in fact advanced when the discussion about the link between smoking and lung cancer began. Therefore person-based studies like those described in Sect. 22.3 were necessary to establish the influence of smoking on lung cancer beyond doubt.

Another example will be presented in Sect. 25.3.

A last remark about terminology: Unfortunately some recent large studies utilize the terms "person-based" and "population-based" with a different meaning, not to be made precise here. Hence, beware of wrong interpretations!

24.2 Evaluating an Intervention

As noted before, when trying to evaluate the influence of educational campaigns like those in the five examples at the beginning of the preceding section, we are in the realm of *experimental* epidemiology because the factors had been created by the health system. This is true for any type of "intervention" in a community. In addition to education, there are indeed many other forms of intervention with the aim of improving the health situation. Examples where the communities may be communes or districts or even entire provinces include better equipment for Commune Health Stations, better training of their staff, better and more generalized health insurance, efficient garbage removal, building of wells and organizing the participation of people in health activities.

Often several of these measures are combined. There exist "comprehensive" interventions directed at specific problems such as the prevention of cardiovascular disorders, which integrate many kinds of measures (Sect. 23.3). Another example is "comprehensive malaria control" that consists of education, the distribution of insecticide-treated bednets, early case detection, better case management and, if feasible, anopheles control (Sect. 7.2).

Vaccinating a whole community is still another type of intervention. In the first place it is a person-based activity since we are vaccinating individuals, and accordingly we have treated the problem of finding the efficacy of a vaccination scheme by a person-based cohort study; see Sect. 18.2. However, we have already mentioned in Sects. 1.1 and 5.3 the indirect effects of a vaccination campaign due to the reduction of the number of sources of infection; they concern the community as a whole.

The effect of interventions is being investigated in "intervention studies", also called "intervention trials". Let us remark in passing that some authors apply the term "intervention" also to preventive and curative treatments of individual persons so that "intervention trial" becomes synonymous with "clinical trial" but we shall not use that terminology.

Recall once again that the influence of a factor of any kind can be evaluated only by comparison. In a community-based study this would mean that in principle we must compare groups of communities determined by different levels of the factor. In the five examples above, we ought to compare some communities where the education campaign was conducted with others where it was not. This is not easy to do in practice. In theory, the Health Department could decide to start the campaign only in some communes but not in others, and then to follow up all communes. This would amount to a community-based cohort study. As in a person-based cohort study, the two "cohorts" of communes would have to be selected by a correct sampling plan in order to make sure that they do not distinguish themselves by another factor that could also influence the outcome. For example, it should not happen that the communes where the campaign is launched are close to the capital whereas the majority of the others are situated far away from it.

There is an important "ethical" problem in this cohort approach similar to the one mentioned in Sect. 18.4 for clinical trials. The communes where the campaign is not conducted will feel disadvantaged, and rightly so!

Moreover, the two cohorts will not necessarily be independent because knowledge of the messages of the campaign will usually spread out to communities where it does not take place.

For such reasons interventions are often evaluated with "historical controls". One compares the situation after the intervention with that before. The problem is, then, the same as in person-based studies. Indeed, other conditions, for example economic ones, may have changed during the period from before to after the intervention and exert an influence that would be hard to separate from the influence of the intervention.

Another difficulty when trying to evaluate an intervention through a community study concerns the outcome. We are rarely satisfied with the simple dichotomy "the health situation has improved or has not improved", that is a binary outcome variable. We are interested in a more complete and detailed description of the changes that may have taken place as a result of the intervention. This is often hard to quantify.

Thus the type of evaluation that appears most appropriate depends very much on the particular situation. The selected evaluation will often be approximate and not very rigorous. In general it cannot be resumed in a single number. Qualitative and to a large extent subjective judgements play an important role.

Nevertheless interventions should not be started without some evidence about their efficacy based on more or less rigorous investigations. This principle is part of what is called "evidence-based public health". It is the analogue to "evidence-based medicine" stated in Sect. 18.3, namely the requirement that all curative and preventive treatments should first be evaluated by a rigorous clinical trial.

24.3   Practical Work

1. In the province of Hà Tinh there is an ongoing educational campaign for better nutrition. Inform yourself about it and analyze it under the following aspects:

   – Quality of the messages.
   – Definition of the outcomes.
   – Possibilities for evaluation.

2. Read and comment critically some reports on community studies that have appeared in the literature.

Lesson 25
Nutritional and Environmental Epidemiology

This is a short glimpse at two areas that are both classical and of high current interest.

25.1 History

Traditional curricula in Public Health contain courses on "Nutrition and Food Safety" and "Environmental Health". In the present lesson we shall show that it is the epidemiologic aspect of these fields that counts in Public Health.

Why treating both subject areas in the same lesson? The answer to this question is simple. Environmental factors act on the human body from outside and nutritional factors from inside. This somewhat superficial statement allows us to structure the presentations of the two fields in a similar way.

The outcome variables in both nutritional and environmental epidemiology are the usual ones: appearance or presence of a given disease or syndrome in an individual; death; various other aspects of health. Hence we are mainly dealing with indicators of the type "incidence", "prevalence" and "mortality". We are interested in the action of nutritional and environmental factors on them.

A distinctive trait of nutritional epidemiology is that almost *all* health outcomes are influenced in some way, directly or indirectly by the diet people are eating. Environmental factors also act on a very large variety of diseases.

In Sect. 1.5 we had put nutritional risk factors into the category "life style" whereas environmental factors form a category of their own. Both are of course also connected with socio-economic factors. Wealthy people eat differently from poor ones although it may not always be healthier. They are also able to influence their environment, for example by living in a less polluted part of the city or in a better house. Hence, confounding is an especially important issue in studies within our two fields. In a survey in 1936 in England it turned out that slum dwellers who had been re-housed to better accommodations had a higher mortality than those who

© Springer Nature Switzerland AG 2019
K. Krickeberg et al., *Epidemiology*, Statistics for Biology and Health,
https://doi.org/10.1007/978-3-030-16368-6_25

continued to live in their slum area because they now had to pay more for rent and had less money left for food.

Let us start with *nutritional epidemiology*. A few more short historical remarks and examples may cast some light on the problems to be treated. Leaving apart the special domains of "food control" and "poisoning", this field has been dealing until recently above all with the influence of *lacking* ingredients of food and of *undernourishment*. Questions of *overnourishment* came up later with rising economic standards. They are now of capital importance in Vietnam, too, although undernourishment persists in some areas and some strata of the population.

Methods for rigorous studies of all forms of wrong diets have been developed mostly over the last 25 years but there were precursors. In 1747 James Lind of the Royal Navy of England showed that "scurvy" is due to the lack of certain ingredients of citrus fruits. He did so by what we now call a clinical trial (Lesson 18). The treatments to be compared were given to the same persons but at different times, namely to 12 sailors suffering from scurvy. He gave them six different supplements to their basic diet, one after the other, and found that citrus fruits, and only these, cured them. By now we know of course that the lacking ingredient was Vitamin C.

The discovery of vitamins and other micronutrients started in the period around 1900, at first mainly based on observations on animals. A long series of investigations led to the realization that the principal factor underlying "beriberi" was a lack of Thiamine, also called Vitamin B_1. The term "vitamin" was coined in 1911 during this string of studies. It had started in 1887 with a comparative study in the Japanese Navy. There, the incidence and mortality by beriberi was high among sailors who ate only polished rice whereas it was low among those who were given in addition fish, meat and vegetables.

Already in 1849 it was discovered in France that cod-liver oil was very effective against "rickets", which carries the scientific name "rachitis". However, it took until the 1920s to clear up the role of Vitamin D deficiency as the main factor. Let us also recall the role of Vitamin A in preventing "xerophthalmia" and other eye problems.

Later on, many other types of micronutrients, in particular minerals, were investigated; see for example Sect. 6.3 for zinc. Every medical student knows the effects of iodine deficiency, namely goitre and often also mental impairment. The same is true for fluorides and caries. A more recent Chinese study showed that selenium deficiency is responsible for a high incidence of the "Keshan disease", a particular cardiomyopathy where a virus may also be involved.

The pathogenic role of general undernourishment as opposed to the lack of specific ingredients has of course been the subject of innumerably many studies. They started essentially around the middle of the nineteenth century. For a long time, they were mainly dealing with the risk factor "energy uptake": how many calories did the members of the target population consume daily? The outcomes of interest were the susceptibility to infectious diseases such as tuberculosis, pneumonia, measles and diarrhoea but also broader outcomes like general morbidity and mortality from all causes, child mortality and deficient health and lower educational achievements of children. More recently, the factor "breastfeeding" was studied.

Overnourishment as a risk factor is a much newer topic and so is imbalanced nutrition in general. Although excessive alcohol and protein consumption have been suspected for centuries to play a role in the aetiology of "gout", in the recent past the issue of overnourishment has taken overwhelming dimensions in many countries including Vietnam.

Overweight and obesity form its visible facet. The most important specific outcomes that have been investigated are type 2 diabetes mellitus, cancer and cardiovascular diseases. Nutritional risk factors for the latter two diseases were already discussed in Sects. 22.3 and 23.2; diabetes will be taken up in the next paragraph. There are in fact only very few health outcomes for which the influence of nutrition has not been suspected or even confirmed. Among those of some importance in Vietnam let us mention, in addition to those just recalled, arthrosis (often also named osteoarthritis), osteoporosis, cataracts, chronic respiratory diseases and even congenital malformations. A typical feature of these outcomes is that in general the influence of imbalanced diet becomes visible only after a long time in contrast to the effect of specific deficiencies. This influences the form of studies to be done.

For type 2 diabetes, risk factors of the category "life style" and in particular nutrition play an overwhelming role. It has turned out that wrong diet and obesity but also lack of physical exercise, stress and certain medications such as glucocorticoïds contribute strongly to the appearance and evolution of the disease. Therefore, differences and changes in life style may explain differences in the situation and trends of the disease between various countries. Roughly speaking, in the USA and, to a lesser degree, in Europe the prevalence density has been high and steadily rising for many years. In China and Vietnam it has been augmenting rapidly in a more recent past. It should also be noted that both changing life styles and higher life expectancies account for a change in the role of the factor "age". Type 2 diabetes mellitus used to be a disease of older people, in general over 40, in contrast to type 1 diabetes mellitus. Now the age of onset decreases, most likely because of a change of eating habits among the young. The presence of more people of high age also leads to higher prevalence.

Environmental factors have been playing a prominent role in medical writings from their beginnings on. They were considered an important part of the aetiology of diseases. Some of them appear in the Chinese Mavangdui texts mentioned in Sect. 15.3. In his treatise "On airs, water, and place" the Greek physician Hippocrates wrote around 400 BC about atmospheric conditions and "*miasmata*" (plural of *miasma*: dirt). Almost 600 years later another Greek physician, Galenos, whose writings have influenced if not dominated European medical thinking well into the nineteenth century, stated that there are three causes of an "epidemic constitution" in a population: susceptibility, life style and atmospheric causes. This is not very far from our present list of categories of risk factors in Sect. 1.5 if we interpret "atmospheric causes" as environmental ones. Specific environmental risk factors related to an occupational disease of miners were described in the sixteenth century in Central Europe. More than 300 years later it turned out that one of the factors was radon and the outcome lung cancer. There was also the famous study by Percival Pott in 1775 in England on the risk of scrotal cancer among chimney sweeps (see Sect. 22.2). However, as said before, in this book we do not treat occupational diseases.

In the nineteenth century we have the study by John Snow of the environmental factor "water" already described in Sect. 6.2.

Industrialization brought many new sources of pollution of the environment and hence many studies followed. Again, tuberculosis was an important outcome. We shall pursue this line in Sect. 25.3.

25.2   Modern Methods in Nutritional Epidemiology

We shall be dealing with malnutrition both in the sense of under- and overnourishment and of an imbalanced diet.

One of the main concerns of present day studies in nutritional epidemiology is to make precise the meaning of exposure variables such as *nutrients, food, diet* and *nutritional status*.

This is not easy. For example it would be wrong to rely on anthropometric measures like weight, height, wasting and stunting to describe the nutritional status of a child. In modern nutritional epidemiology one investigates above all a set of exposure variables that represents *food intake*. From food intake we can derive *dietary patterns*. There have been attempts to summarize food intake by a single variable called "healthy eating index". This amounts, like any single index, to a big loss of information but has some minor practical advantages.

We must also distinguish between *current* food intake, observed at a given moment, and *usual* intake. The latter is of course more interesting to study because we normally expect that it is the eating habits of people in the long run which influence their health. Sometimes investigators simply assume that current intake is more or less typical for usual intake. The appropriate exposure variables also depend on the type of study that we are planning. In a cross-sectional or case–control study one observes in the first place current intake. Information about usual intake relies on the memory of the subjects. In a prospective cohort study usual intake can be measured directly but as said in Sect. 17.2, it is a slow and expensive enterprise.

In any study we have to measure the values of the exposure variables for the individuals involved in accordance with their definition. For current food intake one often asks open-ended questions like: "Tell me what you are eating habitually". In this way one gets a good picture of food consumption but it is hard and slow to evaluate the study because many expected and unexpected answers are possible. For usual food intake, a standard "Food Frequency Questionnaire" exists with coded possible answers.

Given the variety of problems, practically all types of studies are being employed. Some are experimental like Lind's classical trial or the community trials that led to evaluating the influence of fluorides on caries. Most are observational, though; current or usual food intake is a given entity to be observed but not to be influenced by the investigator. We shall not enter into technical details because they depend too much on the specific problems and on the resources available for the investigation.

Finally, let us add a few words about the impact of nutritional epidemiology on disease prevention. Potentially, it is enormous but it depends on political realities. Public health authorities that are trying to further healthier diets by educational campaigns have little power against overwhelming publicity by strong producers of food of doubtful value. This is particularly striking in a country like Vietnam whose traditional food is on the whole quite balanced and healthy in addition to being very tasty and often cheaper. Schools, Commune Health Stations, District Health Centres, Provincial Health Departments, the Ministry of Health, the press, television etc. need to be provided with solid arguments in order to enable them to advocate and pursue an "evidence-based policy" in the domain of nutrition. This must be founded on rigorous and comprehensive studies. Then, in order to convince the population of the necessity of healthy nutrition, efficient methods of health education and health communication are required.

25.3 Modern Methods in Environmental Epidemiology

As we have noted at the beginning of this lesson a short discussion of environmental epidemiology may run more or less along the same lines as the preceding one on nutritional epidemiology. A very large number of health-related outcome variables are being influenced by environmental factors. In present-day Vietnam the most prominent outcomes are cancer and respiratory diseases, both acute and chronic, but also cardiovascular diseases. Allergies and other autoimmune diseases play an increasing role as well. Recently diseases connected with changes of the human hormone system appear more and more.

Before passing to environmental risk factors, let us quote a definition of the environment from a dictionary of epidemiology:

Environment is all that which is external to the human host.

Thus environmental risk factors include infective microorganisms but their study forms a field apart, which we have treated in previous lessons (Lessons 4–10). There are other *biological* risk factors, in particular pollen that may cause allergies. *Physical* risk factors of current interest are radiations, electromagnetic fields, vibrations, noise and heat. Dust and soot, both indoors and outdoors, and asbestos and mineral fibres in buildings may still be counted among physical factors. The weather and climate and especially the ongoing largely man-made climate change will no doubt exert a strong influence on health.

It is likely, though, that the rapidly increasing and largely uncontrolled presence of *chemical* risk factors exerts the greatest pernicious influence on health. They are found everywhere, indoors and outdoors, in the air, soil and water. They stem from industry and traffic, from the use of chemicals in building material and in many modern products sold to the population, from herbicides, pesticides and over-use of fertilizers in agriculture, from waste deposits, but also from forest fires and from passive smoking, which means inhaling the smoke of other people. Many of them are hormone disrupters. Vietnam is being flooded by plastic material; much of it is now known to be harmful to health.

In general the influence of a specific environmental factor on health outcomes is being identified gradually, starting form informal observations like those on radon cited in Sect. 25.1. Preliminary toxicological experiments in vitro or on animals often give a clue to an effect of an agent on health. As in nutritional epidemiology, the "exposure assessment", which means defining the risk factors to be investigated precisely and stating practical rules for measuring them, is a difficult task.

There exist some typical traits of the action of the environment on health that determine the suitable types of studies to be employed. They are:

Environmental exposures are mostly weak but long lasting. Risks and risk ratios are small. There exist many confounding factors.

We have already looked at some examples in Sects. 22.3 and 23.2. The fact that the risks in exposed and non-exposed populations are small implies that cohort studies are long and expensive and require large sample sizes; in fact, relatively few have been conducted. Case–control studies are more frequent; we have indeed observed in Sect. 20.2 that they are well adapted to situations where the risks are small. However, they require assessing exposures in cases and controls retrospectively, which may not always be possible.

Early environmental epidemiology has sometimes used community studies but their results are often of limited interest because they may suffer from the ecological fallacy (Sect. 24.1). In order to let the basic idea of an ecological fallacy in environmental epidemiology come out clearly, we are going to construct a simplified fictitious example. Suppose that in a cross-sectional ecological study we compare a few cities regarding their average sulphur dioxide concentration in the air during the year 2015 and we also register, for each city, the reported incidence density of asthmatic crises during that year. Suppose now that the cities with a higher sulphur dioxide exposure have, on the whole, a lower relative incidence of asthmatic crises. Does this mean that sulphur dioxide in the air protects against asthmatic crises? Not necessarily so. The sulphur dioxide concentration within a city varies a lot due to winds, the relief, the presence of high or low buildings etc. We can imagine that in some cities the high overall concentration of SO_2 in the air is due to very high concentrations in a few industrial districts counting few residents whereas the majority of inhabitants live in parts of the city where the air is relatively clean. By contrast, in cities with low overall concentration of SO_2 this concentration may be more evenly distributed and affect most everybody, which would explain the phenomenon described above. Suppose, finally, that in a sample survey we are able to look at individual data. Then it may very well turn out that subjects with a higher exposure *do* in fact have a higher risk of an asthmatic crisis.

Let us come to the role of environmental epidemiology in disease prevention. We could say almost the same as for nutritional epidemiology, with obvious modifications. In Vietnam the impact on health of environmental factors is rapidly becoming a problem of highest importance. It is a political problem concerning mainly economic policy. Health authorities are still too weak to resist pressure from industry and other sectors of the economy that consider questions of the environment mainly from the point of view of immediate cost and profit to them. Again, we can quote active and passive smoking as a typical example. It belongs both to the category "life style" and "environmental factors". We have discussed its effect on various types of cancer in Sects. 22.2 and 22.3 and on cardio-vascular diseases in Sect. 23.2. It is also the main cause of another severe disease of rapidly growing prevalence in Vietnam, namely *chronic obstructive bronchitis*. Measures by public health authorities against smoking are still inadequate. The same can be said about many other environmental risks.

25.4 Practical Work

1. Design a simple questionnaire for a survey on *current* and *usual* food intake in your commune. Decide yourself about the questions to be included.
2. Plan and conduct a small survey in your neighbourhood on *changes* in food intake during the last 5 years.
3. On the basis of what you have heard and read about the influence of nutritional factors on health, review traditional eating in your province critically. What should be reduced or eliminated, what should be added?
4. What are, in your opinion, the principal environmental risk factors in your vicinity? Which type of study would you use in order to investigate their impact?

Lesson 26
Social and Genetic Epidemiology

These are two modern and rapidly developing fields that have important actual and potential applications in Public Health.

26.1 Factors and the History of their Study

In Sect. 1.5 we have listed the main categories of factors that may influence health. The "classical" factors age, sex, time and place are the subject of purely descriptive epidemiology, which is a century-old area that started with registries of causes of death. The other categories of the list have been studied systematically only in a more recent past, and that was the beginning of modern epidemiology.

In the present lesson we shall have a closer look at the categories "social and economic conditions" and "genetic factors". The study of their influence on health is called "Social Epidemiology" and "Genetic Epidemiology", respectively. In spite of a very different historical development, these two fields have in common that they are at present the subject of particularly intensive interest and research. They have already had important applications in Public Health and will undoubtedly play a prominent role in the future. They are also tied to each other by contrasts. Essentially, genetic factors are created by nature while social ones are made by man. Genetic factors can rarely be observed directly. Normally one observes the outcome in the first place, and hence the typical study is "case-control" although often in a more refined and complex form. In social epidemiology, one starts from social conditions and the ideal study type is, therefore, to follow cohorts.

In order to simplify the language, we shall write "social" when we mean "social and economic", thus including economic factors among social ones. In social epidemiology the term "determinant" is commonly being used instead of "factor" or "exposure variable".

Examples of the influence of social and genetic factors have already appeared in many places in this book. The gentle reader may want to go back to the sections where they can be found. Thus, social determinants of health came up for occupational diseases (Sect. 22.3), cholera (Sect. 6.2), tuberculosis (Sects. 7.2 and

© Springer Nature Switzerland AG 2019
K. Krickeberg et al., *Epidemiology*, Statistics for Biology and Health,
https://doi.org/10.1007/978-3-030-16368-6_26

21.1), dengue fever (Sect. 8.4), HIV/AIDS (Sect. 10.4), cancer (Sect. 22.3), cardio-vascular diseases (Sect. 23.2) and in a general way at the end of Sect. 24.1. Genetic factors appeared for tuberculosis (Sect. 7.2), malaria (Sect. 7.2), dengue fever (Sect. 8.4), cancer (Sect. 22.3), and cardiovascular diseases (Sect. 23.2).

The role of *social* risk factors was recognized long ago. The risks of specific dangerous occupations were already mentioned in antiquity and studied more closely from the sixteenth century on. However, we shall not treat these factors here because they are largely not so much social factors but factors of physical environ-ment or life style; "Occupational Diseases" is a field of its own. We shall focus on social determinants in the narrower sense of social inequality, income and poverty including housing conditions, social standing, education etc. They are also called "vertical" social factors. More recently determinants such as social networks were defined and investigated.

Vertical factors imply the idea of a social hierarchy. The general theme is, for example: "Are poorer people in worse health than rich ones"?

It was already known in the middle ages that leprosy is particularly endemic among the poor. In 1848 the comprehensive "Report on the sanitary condition of the labouring population of Great Britain" by the lawyer and civil servant Edwin Chadwick appeared. In the same year the physician Rudolf Virchow published a report on an epidemic of louse-born typhus in a peripheral region of Germany in which he pointed out major social risk factors. He stressed the dreadful influence of general backwardness, poverty and lack of education and freedom. His later propos-als for central water supply and faeces disposal in the city of Berlin were speedily executed. Chadwick, Virchow and a few others at about the same time became pio-neers of "Social Medicine". They wrote:

"Medicine is a social science"

and Virchow added:

"Politics is nothing but medicine on a large scale".

The term "social medicine" remained a bit vague. For some people it amounted to the study of social determinants of health and its applications, that is, to social epidemiology in the sense of the present Lesson. For others it was tantamount to Public Health but there the term "Social Hygiene"soon prevailed; see Sect. 29.1.

Chadwick and Virchow did not yet conduct a comparative study in the modern sense. These began in many countries in the second half of the nineteenth century. Most of them were, in modern terminology, record-based retrospective cohort stud-ies that used registries from hospitals, health insurances and declarations of causes of death. Some studies were person-based and others were community studies. All the vertical factors listed above were investigated. Regarding the outcome variables, infectious diseases and in particular tuberculosis and sexually transmitted diseases played a prominent role, but also nervous and mental illness, tumours and dental decay. On the whole, the pernicious influence of the social factors in question was confirmed. In the beginning of the twentieth century the study of social determinants of health was already a well-established discipline that employed fairly modern concepts such as for example "confounding", which was called "veiling", and "bias". A comprehensive treatise in German of 880 pages entitled "Disease and social condition" appeared in 1913; it is still being reprinted. A large part of that book was devoted to possible interventions, especially by the state.

By now the influence of social inequality on health has been investigated in many developing and developed countries and for most major diseases. In general it has turned out that people of lower social status are indeed less healthy and have a higher mortality and lower life expectancy. In the next section we shall look into the basic ideas and methods and present some recent examples, touching also on non-vertical factors.

The history of *genetic* epidemiology is much younger. True, the vague idea of a "predisposition" or "susceptibility" of a person for a given disease has always existed and people have speculated about whether it may be hereditary or not. Leprosy and tuberculosis were typical examples but also breast cancer, diabetes and epilepsy. However, a rigorous study of these questions could not start before the main tools of genetic epidemiology had been sufficiently developed.

The basic tools of genetic epidemiology are population genetics and molecular genetics.

They had not reached maturity before the second half of the twentieth century in spite of early beginnings with Gregor Mendel's laws in 1866.

The risk factors in genetic epidemiology are the existence of particular genes and combinations of genes that raise the probability of the appearance of given health problems. They are being described and their action is being studied by combining methods of population genetics and molecular genetics.

In *population genetics* we would ask: "Has the disease appeared or existed in the family of the patient?" This needs of course to be made precise: where and when did it appear in the family? Population genetics is to a large extent a mathematical–statistical tool. We shall give here an example that is already almost "historical", dating from the year 1989 and concerning leprosy. By analyzing the family links between individuals suffering from this disease it was shown that the susceptibility to leprosy is indeed hereditary. In order to exclude influences from outside the target population, the investigators conducted the study in a "closed" population, namely on an island in the Caribbean. Similar studies followed, for example in southern Vietnam in 1995. By now, using methods of molecular genetics, one has also identified the genes associated with leprosy.

We have already sketched at the end of Sect. 7.2 an earlier example based on observations but not on a rigorous study. In 1949 it became known, from a rudimentary reasoning of population genetics, that sickle cell anaemia is a "hereditary" disease. Later, the mutation at the root of sickle cell anaemia was found. Persons who carry this mutation in a heterozygous form, that is, on one chromosome only, are less susceptible to malaria than persons without this mutation; if infected the disease takes a milder course. Persons afflicted with the homozygous form of the mutation have a very low life expectancy.

Finally, we mention a classical example, namely Down's syndrome, also called trisomy 21; an obsolete name is mongolism. In 1959 it was discovered that it is the result of the presence of an extra chromosome 21 or of part of it. It is rarely hereditary; the chromosomal abnormality of the child is due to a genetic change prior to conception of the egg cell of the mother or, in about one tenth of all cases, the sperm of the father.

In *molecular genetics* we ask: what is the molecular structure of our genes and how does it influence their function?

26.2   Modern Studies in Social Epidemiology

The general theme of modern social epidemiology is well defined. It is the study of the influence on health of social factors that represent social inequalities. It comprises practical conclusions, above all recommendations to health authorities and governments, but also to the population.

As everywhere in epidemiology, what we have to do before starting a study is to make precise the underlying ideas and concepts:

- Which target population do we have in mind?
- What are the outcome variables of interest?
- What are the social risk factors that ought to be studied?
- How do we describe best the influence of the latter on the former?
- Which types of study are appropriate?
- How can we interpret the results, for example in the form of hints to causal relations?
- Which useful practical conclusions can be drawn?

Regarding *target populations*, social inequalities exist in most groups of people, and so there is a large variety of human populations that have been investigated. Many studies are "person-based", that is, the social determinants and the health-related outcome variables are defined for individual persons. However, it is characteristic for social epidemiology that "community-based" concepts and methods (Sect. 24.1) play an important and ever-increasing role. As remarked above, this started already in the late nineteenth century and early twentieth century and the trend continues. Typical communities are villages, cities, communes, provinces and countries but they may also be defined in many other ways, for example by profession.

It is fairly clear what the *outcome variables* of interest will be. In a person-based approach the classical outcomes to be measured for individual persons are the occurrence or presence of a specific disease such as tuberculosis, death from a given disease and death from any cause. Accordingly one is interested in the influence of social determinants on indicators such as incidence or prevalence of a disease, mortality by a given disease, mortality from all causes, infant mortality, life-expectancy and the like. These outcome variables and indicators still play a predominant role in modern investigations but several more have entered the scene. They concern characteristics of health such as fitness for work, disabilities and various subjective appreciations of "being well".

As observed in Sect. 24.1, in a community-based approach the value of an outcome variable for a given community is almost always derived from a person-based variable by forming an average. This is in particular true for all examples there; the reader should have another look at them.

For risk factors, in other words *determinants*, to which we are turning now, the situation is quite different. We have mentioned the traditional vertical social risk factors in the preceding section: income, poverty or wealth, housing, social standing and education. Many old and new studies are person-based as in the examples quoted there. However, community-based determinants appear already in some studies from the late nineteenth century. Most of them are still obtained from person-based factors by averaging, for example average income or number of people having received secondary education. Let us quote a slightly more bizarre example. In 1911 the report on a community study appeared which compared districts (*arrondissements*) of Paris with each other. The risk factor was "number of windows per person" and the outcome was "mortality rate from tuberculosis from 1858 to 1902". The influence of this factor was striking; the higher the average number of windows the lower the mortality by tuberculosis.

A typical trait of modern social epidemiology is the growing number of issues that are influenced by newer developments within the field of sociology. In particular this means that more and more community-based determinants appear that cannot be derived from person-based ones. They concern social structures within a community that may be resumed under headings like "social networks", "social environment", "social support" and "social capital". In order to study their influence on health, they need to be defined in a quantitative way.

One of the main problems of contemporary social epidemiology is the rigorous quantitative definition of risk factors that represent social structures.

We shall illustrate this below by some examples.

Turning to the next topic listed above, namely investigating the *influence* of social risk factors on various health outcome variables, we arrive at another basic issue of modern social epidemiology, namely the analysis of "pathways".

A pathway in a study consists of the chain of events from an exposition to the outcome.

In order to illustrate the concept let us look at the "first Whitehall study" in Great Britain, which started in 1967. The target population consisted of civil servants. Their social status was defined by their employment grade on an official scale. The study revealed a very strong influence of the factor "low grade" on general mortality and on mortality by cardiovascular diseases. When we describe matters within the epidemiologic set-up presented in Sect. 15.1 this means that civil servants of lower grades have a higher probability of dying than those in higher grades; this is in fact true in all age-groups, even after retirement.

But why is this so? The social grade hardly influences *directly* the probability of dying; there are intermediate steps that form a pathway from the exposure to the outcome. Let us speculate on some *conceivable* pathways.

One of the last steps of a pathway is always the action of certain biological variables that may lead directly to illness and death. They include abnormal hormone values or blood counts, wrong immune responses, latent infections etc., generally on the sub-clinical level. Their influence can be modified by medical interventions, both preventive and curative. This fact suggests a first possible pathway: subjects of lower social status have less access to good health care, which influences the action of various pathogenic factors, which in turn bears on mortality.

However, it has been shown that this is not the only, and not even the most important pathway, especially in countries with fairly evenly distributed quality of health care. A second conceivable pathway that has attracted much attention passes through the factor "stress". A low social position may produce stress in many ways, directly by work pressure but also because of frustration, lack of recognition or fewer social contacts. The next step, the influence of stress on the biological variables has been the subject of many psychological and sociological studies.

A third pathway can be imagined via behaviour. People of lower social status are perhaps more inclined to adopt an unwholesome life style such as excessive alcohol consumption, smoking, unhealthy nutrition, irregular sleeping hours, lack of physical exercise or just "not taking care of themselves". Combinations and interactions of these pathways may also intervene, for example lower social status leads to stress, which in turn results in an unwholesome life style. However, the actual role of these possible pathways has only been investigated for very few of them. A graphical representation of all sorts of pathways that can be imagined is sometimes called a "model" for the action of social determinants.

The next question on our list above was: What *types of study* are appropriate? Let us first consider person-based studies. Register-based retrospective cohort studies as in the "classical" period before the First World War still appear but their scope is limited because only few vertical social factors are recorded in registers such as those for admission to hospitals or death registers. For example in Great Britain the profession of a deceased person is indicated on the death certificate; in Vietnam and Germany it is not. For the same reason case–control studies are rarely feasible because it is in most situations impossible to determine the social status of the patient in a case of a disease or death.

The ideal but slow and expensive type of study in social epidemiology is a prospective cohort study.

In such studies cohorts are defined by different levels of social factors. They are being followed over time and the outcome is measured. In the first Whitehall study the cohorts of civil servants determined by employment grades were followed over 25 years.

Community-based studies need to be done if the risk factors are only defined for communities, not for individual persons. The second of the three examples below is of this type. Community studies are particularly appropriate in countries with good statistical capabilities where social indicators about administrative units are available.

The last but first question, namely the *interpretation* of the results, in particular in view of causal relations, is intimately connected with the question of pathways; there in each step, the question of a causal relation appears. Much research is still needed. We shall not pursue this here and only refer to the discussion in Sects. 15.3 and 17.2.

Before commenting the last topic in the list, which may lead to *useful practical conclusions* to the benefit of Public Health, we shall illustrate it by three recent typical examples from Germany, the USA and Vietnam.

In studies after the Second World War, the emphasis was first on cardiovascular diseases and, to a minor degree, cancer as these appeared to be the main health problems of developed countries. Then the interest in infectious diseases rose again as in the "classical" period of social epidemiology; tuberculosis became the focus of attention once more and finally AIDS.

In an industrialized country like Germany where the overall morbidity by tuberculosis has been low during the last four decades or so the influence of special vertical social factors such as *migration* is a particularly interesting subject. In a community-based study in the city of Cologne with about one million residents that was published in 2002, 78 sub-districts of the city were compared. The value of the outcome variable for such a community was defined as the annual incidence rate of tuberculosis, averaged over the period 1986–1997. This was derived from the declaration of individual cases, which is compulsory. For each community, 12 socio-demographic and socio-economic indicators that were considered possible risk factors could be obtained from statistical offices of the city and health authorities. All of them had been calculated from data about individual subjects. Again, the methods of evaluation were those of a community-based retrospective cohort study. Pathways and causal relationships were also being discussed. We shall only mention two interesting and perhaps unexpected results. High incidence of tuberculosis among migrants from abroad to Cologne was more due to present material deprivation than to former infections before they arrived. The effect of AIDS on tuberculosis incidence still appeared fairly small at that time.

A study in the USA published in 2001 is concerned with the same type of outcome variable derived from recorded cases of tuberculosis in the period 1985–1992. It took place in the state of New Jersey and its purpose was to investigate the influence of social determinants such as "segregation" of ethnic groups in addition to more classical ones like "poverty". There were four ethnic groups: non-Hispanic Whites, African Americans, Hispanics and Asians. The state of New Jersey is divided into 591 areas defined by a common postal code. A "community" was defined to be *one* ethnic group in *one* area, which gives $4 \times 591 = 2264$ communities to be compared. Let us look for example at the risk factor "isolation", which is one aspect of segregation. The "degree of isolation within a community" is an example of a risk factor that is not derived from a person-based variable by averaging. It concerns indeed a social structure, that is, relations *between several* individuals of a community, namely contacts of individuals with members of the same ethnic group in the same area. The precise quantitative definition is a bit complicated and will not be given here.

This study is also interesting and original in another respect. Although in the first place cross-sectional, it is evaluated like a generalized case–control study; see the discussion after the 2 × 2-table in Sect. 19.2. The results point to a detrimental influence on tuberculosis incidence of the risk factors studied, in particular isolation, among African Americans but isolation seemed to have on the contrary a protective effect among non-Hispanic Whites.

Until now, not many rigorous studies in social epidemiology were conducted in Vietnam. Given the fast socio-economic changes that are taking place in the country, the subject is of capital importance, though, for planning the health system and for decisions about health strategies. We are going to review a relatively simple cross-sectional survey published in 2006. As in the two preceding examples it stresses certain social risk factors that have been in the centre of interest of more recent sociological research in contrast to classical factors like income, wealth, education and social status. These factors are person-based and represent aspects of social capital.

The target population consisted of mothers and their 1 year old or 8 years old children in five provinces of Vietnam. The "social capital" factors concerned the mothers and the outcome variables described aspects of the health of their children. Social capital has a "structural" component defined by active participation in groups such as the Women's Union, trade unions or private groups and by support from social networks. It also has a "cognitive", subjective component defined by what mothers think about their social surroundings, for example whether they can trust most people in their commune. Both components are measured in quantitative terms by putting questions to the mothers. The health of their children, too, was defined by the answers of their mothers to certain questions about illnesses in a recent past. For example one of these questions was, for 8 years old children: "Has your child suffered from a life threatening disease in the past 3 years?"

In contrast to the two preceding studies this one employed sampling. It used a two-stage sampling plan; see Sect. 12.2. First, 20 "sites" were selected that consisted each of one or two communes. Then a sample of children was drawn from every site, which gave a sample of 2000 one year old and of 1000 eight years old children. With a few exceptions, their mothers were interviewed by questionnaires. The resulting data of this cross-sectional survey were evaluated as in a cohort study. Recall now from Sect. 17.1 that this means comparing indicators derived from outcome variables between groups of mothers determined by different values of the risk factors. For example, is an incidence lower among children of mothers who trust most people in their commune than among children of mothers who do not? We shall not enter into the technical details but resume the main results. High social support and large cognitive social capital of mothers do indeed lead to better health of their children. Active participation in social groups, however, does not seem to have such an effect.

Let us stress that these results are of a purely statistical nature. The question of pathways and causal relations remains open. Does social support or cognitive social capital lead to a better use of health services? Or do they imply that the mother takes better care of her children? Or do they result in better health of the mother, which, in turn, influences the health of her children favourably? Or do they act on the health of the children because they provide a better income to the family? To answer these questions, other studies including prospective cohort studies are needed.

Conclusions from the findings of studies in social epidemiology are often easy to draw and to transform into recommendations to health authorities and governments. Their implementation is another matter. It is clear that:

Implementing recommendations based on results in social epidemiology usually requires an economic foundation but also, and more importantly, political will.

A list of recommendations was given in the final report (2008) of the "Commission on Social Determinants of Health" set up by WHO, available at <www.who.int/social_determinants/en>.

26.3   Modern Studies in Genetic Epidemiology

Genetic epidemiology is a new field. It requires advanced tools from population genetics and molecular genetics with which the reader may not be sufficiently acquainted. However, in principle we are again faced with the questions formulated at the beginning of the preceding section.

- Target populations: Any human population. "Natural" populations to be studied would be the entire world population (even though we can only draw a small sample from it!), a geographical region, for example an island, or an ethnic group. Populations defined by arbitrary man-made boundaries like cities, provinces and countries are also the object of interest, usually because they are easier to study.
- Outcome variables: As in other branches of epidemiology they represent originally the occurrence or the presence or the course of a specific disease *in an individual*. Variables defined from the beginning for communities do hardly occur. Modern genetic epidemiology increasingly investigates outcomes that are only indirectly observable. It does so with the help of "biological markers". This makes it possible to include diseases that have no clear-cut clinical definition such as Crohn's disease (*Enteritis regionalis*) and those that pass through several phases which are difficult to distinguish clinically like breast cancer; for the latter the oestrogen receptor status is being used as outcome.
- Genetic risk factors: In principle, any "genome", that is, the complete set of an individual's genetic material. Naturally, one is much interested in genomes that are in some sense "abnormal", often due to a mutation; at the end of Sect. 26.1 we have mentioned the classical example of trisomy 21. It is again typical for modern genetic epidemiology that the risk factors, too, when they cannot be observed directly, are replaced by biological markers, for example by various agents in the blood.

In genetic epidemiology, one often represents outcomes and risk factors by biological markers.

- Describing the influence of genetic risk factors on the outcome: In principle, looking back to Sect. 15.1, all we have to do is to indicate, for any genome, the probability for the possible values of the outcome variables under consideration, for example the probability that a person with a given genome develops leprosy during her or his lifetime. This probability is called the "penetrance" of the genome towards the outcome in question. It is a precise way of describing the old concept of the predisposition of persons to certain diseases, also known as "susceptibility". As before, modern genetic epidemiology often represents the susceptibility by a proxy in the form of a biological marker.
- Appropriate study types: Many forms of studies are being employed, some of them very involved, but for the sake of clarity and by simplifying a bit we shall repeat what we have said before:

Basically, case-control studies are the natural way of investigating in genetic epidemiology.

Let us now have a closer look at these issues with the help of a few examples. Usually, informal observations of the distribution of a disease motivate more rigorous investigations. To have something concrete in mind let us think of "diabetes mellitus of type 2", which also used to be called non-insulin dependent diabetes mellitus. It may not be a perfect first example because its aetiology is very complex but it is considered an epidemic in developed countries and is rapidly increasing in Vietnam (see Sect. 25.1). An informal observation of the kind just mentioned is that in identical twins, if one of the two siblings has it, the other one has it with a probability around 3/4. This suggests the existence of a genetic component.

After initial observations of this kind that consist in looking at "family histories" of the disease, two kinds of rigorous studies can be distinguished according to the two types of tools mentioned in Sect. 26.1. The first tool is *population genetics*:

Human population genetics is the science of the statistical distribution of alleles (the various possible forms of a gene) in human populations and of their evolution.

Applying population genetics to studies in genetic epidemiology means in particular to carry out a so-called "segregation analysis". For example, a sample consisting of families including several generations is taken and the cases are being recorded together with the "genealogy", that is, the structure of the families. Then one can calculate, for various conceivable modes of inheritance of the disease, the probability that existed for obtaining the *observed* pattern of cases. This is done with the help of a "genetic model", which represents in mathematical terms conceivable mechanisms of inheritance. Finally the mechanism of highest probability is considered to be the one that has actually been at work. It may reveal that a specific genetic factor was involved.

This type of study was used in the studies on leprosy sketched above. It works well for diseases that can be clearly diagnosed and are "monogenic", that is, due to a mutation in a single well-determined gene, for example mucoviscidose (cystic fibrosis). Many diseases that carry a high burden in present day Vietnam are not of this type, though. They present a much more complicated picture. It may not be easy to describe them clinically nor to observe them directly. Therefore, modern genetic epidemiology also uses a second tool, namely *molecular genetics*, especially methods based on biological markers. Doing this is sometimes called "molecular epidemiology":

Molecular epidemiology denotes the integration of biological markers into the epidemiological description of exposures, susceptibilities and outcomes.

An additional difficulty results from the fact that the diseases in question are mostly multi-factorial; see Lesson 28. Many genes may act together in addition to factors from the environment and life style. Let us close this section by sketching two examples.

For *type 2 diabetes mellitus*, the contribution of genetic factors is still not completely elucidated. Ethnic origin is one of them. Many studies have compared ethnic groups *within* a given country, for example the USA. There, African Americans, certain native Indians and some Asians seem to be at higher risk than so-called Caucasians. With the help of molecular genetics, several more genes have been identified recently whose variations influence the evolution of the disease.

Studying the *interplay*, or *interaction* (see again Lesson 28) between genetic and life style factors for type 2 diabetes mellitus is far from terminated. Let us just quote one observation. It seems that in China in the recent past obesity contributed to the appearance of the disease more rapidly, that is, already at a lower level, than in the USA. This may be due to the ethnic factor; an alternative explanation that has been advanced is malnutrition of many Chinese infants.

Chronic respiratory diseases such as *asthma* are also rapidly spreading in Vietnam. They could be discussed along the same lines but we shall not do it here.

Genetic factors for certain forms of cancer and for cardiovascular diseases were briefly mentioned in Sect. 21.3 and 23.2, respectively.

26.4   Applications of Genetic Epidemiology

There are two classical areas of applications of genetic epidemiology and three more recent ones:

- Genetic screening.
- Genetic counselling.
- Genetic therapy.
- Predictive medicine.
- Personalized treatment.

Genetic screening is the systematic search for genetic risk factors in a given population by a screening programme of the type defined in Sect. 19.3.

It is sometimes called "genetic testing" but the expression "screening" is better suited for conveying the idea of a systematic search.

Genetic counselling means advising persons at risk for a genetic disorder about its nature and presenting the options open to them and their consequences.

Both genetic screening and genetic counselling employ tests as treated in Sect. 19.2. The second is often done as a consequence of the result of the first. A person may ask for advice either because of the outcome of a screening programme in which she or he has taken part or for other reasons, for example because of her or his family history. The advice given will of course be based on the possible harmful consequences of the existing genetic disorder in question: which harmful effects on the health of the person are to be expected?

Predicting such effects is called "Genetic Prediction". It rests on the evaluation of many known cases analogously to the estimation of the characteristics of a diagnostic test.

Most of the general comments on screening programmes made in Sect. 19.3 apply to genetic screening as well. Thus, before embarking on such a programme, the pros and cons need to be carefully evaluated. Screening makes sense only if, for every "case" detected early, a reasonable and useful course of action can be proposed that is likely to bring along a real benefit. Harmful side effects of the tests that are being used need to be taken into account. It is at the planning stage of a genetic screening programme that knowledge of the epidemiologic characteristics of the genetic disorder at hand is needed.

The tests used in genetic screening and genetic counselling may be prenatal, apply to newborns, or be done later depending on the problem at hand. They concern mostly *inherited* genetic disorders but sometimes also mutant forms of genes that originated later in life. The genetic material to be investigated is taken from the mouth or, in prenatal testing, from the amniotic fluid with the help of a needle. The latter is called an "amniocentesis"; it implies a small risk of miscarriage. Genetic markers in the blood are also being used. A different form of test consists in studying the history of the disease in question in the family of the subject.

Here are a few examples. Prenatal screening by amniocentesis in order to discover a foetus suffering from trisomy 21 started already in the 1960s. As remarked in the preceding section, this genetic condition is rarely inherited. Genetic counselling concerns a possible abortion.

In some regions of the world there is screening by amniocentesis for sickle cell anaemia, which is hereditary; see the end of Sect. 7.2. Genetic counselling is then provided to carriers who intend to have a child.

In several countries it is compulsory to check every newborn for hypothyroidism and phenylketonuria via an appropriate blood test. At this stage there exists an efficient treatment of each of the two conditions, as every medical student will know.

The most widely applied genetic test to be performed later in life that rests on family histories concerns breast cancer; in Vietnam it is being done in speciality clinics. Here, genetic counselling is not easy. It has happened that women resorted to a radical mastectomy on both sides as a preventive measure because of a high risk deduced from cases of breast cancer in the family. A better alternative for them would have been to submit to more intensive screening for early stages of the disease.

Genetic therapy aims at treating a genetic disease by replacing the underlying deleterious gene by another one.

Its epidemiologic components are easy to imagine. They consist in investigating the results of the intervention and in particular possible harmful side effects and their relations with other factors.

The term Predictive Medicine denotes several different subject areas but genetic epidemiology plays a role in all of them, similarly to that played be clinical trials in normal clinical medicine.

Indeed, in its classical form predictive medicine means predicting the evolution of an illness of a particular patient already under treatment for this illness. More recently the concept has been enlarged in fairly vague ways to mean or to include for instance the prediction of such and such illness in a given person not yet suffering from it, or the prediction of certain diseases in a population. Whatever the interpretation of the term may be, genetic information is now frequently included among the input variables. The prediction provides among others the estimated influence of this variable in the particular case being dealt with, and to this end it takes into account the results of previous epidemiologic studies of such an influence in populations.

Personalized Treatment means to determine the treatment of a case on the basis of more detailed knowledge of the patient than usual.

This is of course a very vague definition. Physicians have been applying personalized treatments to different degrees for several millennia. In the recent past the term was mainly used to denote treatments of certain forms of cancer that take into account cancer-associated genes of the patient. The preceding remarks about the necessity of previous studies in genetic epidemiology apply as well.

26.5 Practical Work

1. An exercise in using the medical information base "Medline/Pubmed" (www.pubmed.gov): Search for recent publications under the heading "Social epidemiology, Vietnam". Look at some titles and abstracts that seem interesting to you and try to understand their meaning and relevance. Load down a full paper if it is free. Explore links.

2. The same with "Genetic epidemiology, Vietnam".
3. Plan a cohort study (not to be executed!) in the following setting and give answers to the last two questions:

   - Target population: all adults of a given district who are aged 18–65 years at the beginning of the study (Day 0).
   - Outcome variable: death from any cause during the period between Day 0 and 10 years later.
   - Risk factors: professional status on Day 0. They should be defined by yourself, but include the distinction between "cadre" (cán bô) and "not cadre". Would it be more reasonable to have many or only a few status groups?
   - Evaluation: elementary; compute mortality rates for all professional status groups and compare any two of them along the lines of Sect. 17.1.
   - What would it mean in practical terms to adjust for the factor "rural/urban"? See Sect. 21.2.
   - Would it be of interest to distinguish between the two outcome variables "death from traffic accidents" and "death from illness or other accidents"?
   - Before writing your plan, consult Lesson 27.

4. Try to answer the following question: Why can we not deduce the existence of an ethnic risk factor for type 2 diabetes mellitus by comparing incidence or prevalence densities *between* different countries?

Lesson 27
Some Practical Considerations Around Epidemiologic Studies

The basic ideas of epidemiologic studies were treated in the preceding lessons, both in a general context and within the framework of specific health outcomes or specific risk factors. However, in practice, many details need to be observed.

27.1 Planning the Study

Epidemiologic studies need to be carefully planned before they begin. This is true for any kind of study, be it a simple sample survey, a study of one of the types defined in Sect. 15.2, or a community study as described in Sect. 24.1. The plan of the study, which is also called the "study protocol", must cover all its aspects and stages.

A classical mistake that is still being made from time to time consists in saying: "Let us collect the data first, and then start thinking about how to analyze them". Recall from Sect. 15.3 that the analysis and interpretation of the data depends crucially on the way they had been obtained. The team of investigators needs to define not only the data collection but also the core methods of analysis and evaluation *before* starting the study; they are part of the study plan. This does not exclude another look at the data after the study from a different angle, for example when they seem to point to something unexpected.

In almost all stages of a study there may be systematic errors, in other words a "bias". Hence we shall treat this topic in the special Sects. 27.2 and 27.3. What to do about the various possible forms of bias needs to be said in the study plan.

What else is to be covered by the plan? To start with, the *objectives* must be well defined including the target population, the exposure factors, the outcome variables and their relations. Many examples were given throughout this book. When stating the objectives, it should also be said *why* the study is required and with which degree of *urgency*. This involves in particular a survey of the *existing publications* on the problem at hand.

The *team* of people to conduct the study has to be constituted. In addition to epidemiologists, physicians and health officials who are directly interested in the objectives, this team may include administrators such as the head of the People's Committee of a

© Springer Nature Switzerland AG 2019
K. Krickeberg et al., *Epidemiology*, Statistics for Biology and Health,
https://doi.org/10.1007/978-3-030-16368-6_27

commune, district or province. If one of the special programmes sketched in previous lessons (MCH, EPI, AIDS, …) is concerned, there may be persons who work for them.

The *type of study* is part of the plan. Next, the way of selecting the *study population,* that is the various samples entering the study including their sample size, is to be described in detail. We have sketched this in the relevant lessons.

After that, the plan must indicate how the values of the exposure and outcome variables are to be measured, in other words how the *data* are to be obtained. This will be taken up in Sect. 27.3.

The *analysis* of the data and the interpretation of the results (Sect. 27.4) will normally require a person who knows the relevant mathematical–statistical methods, for example a competent epidemiologist or a mathematical statistician. This person needs to be a member of the study team from the very beginning and has to take part in drawing up all aspects of the planning.

Finally the protocol will say what to do with the results. What kind of report is to be submitted to which services? Is it intended to make recommendations to the population, health officials, politicians etc. if the results seem to suggest it? Should there be a publication about the study and if so, when and where? This will be sketched in Sect. 27.6.

All of these aspects are closely related to, and to a large extent determined by, the question of *funding* the study. The *timeframe* of the study, too, needs to be defined by the plan.

Sometimes it will be reasonable to foresee a *pilot study* on a smaller scale in order to test some of the methods to be employed in the study, in particular in the collection of data. The design of questionnaires may be changed as a result of such a study. There is often also a purely technical reason for doing a pilot study that we have described in detail in Sects. 12.5 and 14.2, namely to obtain *a priori* information required for choosing an appropriate sample size.

In addition to these "obvious" components of the study plan there are some that are occasionally forgotten. In particular *ethical* considerations may determine the form of the study. We have treated this in Sect. 18.5 and shall come back to it in Sect. 27.5.

27.2 Bias

In a scientific and technical context "bias" means a "systematic error" inherent in a measuring device, which persists when the measures are being repeated. It is thus to be distinguished from the "random errors" in single measurements. This idea also underlies the concept of bias in epidemiology.

A bias can arise at several stages of an epidemiologic study. First, there may be a bias when the study population is selected from the target population. Any such bias is called a "selection bias". Next, some types of bias occur when the study population has already been chosen and is being "observed". We shall subsume this under the heading "information bias". There may also be systematic errors in the final statistical analysis but this is rare unless the study team comprises no statistician. Finally, a bias may be caused by the way the results of the study are being disseminated. This is a so-called "publication bias". In brief:

There are three categories of bias: selection bias, information bias and publication bias.

Let us look at details.

A *selection bias* occurs when we sample from the wrong target population or use a bad sampling plan. In Sects. 13.5 and 20.1 we have already mentioned the "hospital bias", which arises when controls are taken only from a hospital whereas the target population consists, for example, of *all* inhabitants of a district. Relying on volunteers for a study also usually causes a selection bias. We may find them through an advertising campaign by mail, e-mail, newspapers, television, posters, telephone or personal contacts but there will always be people who do not respond or do not consent to take part in a given study; thus the volunteers may not be "representative" of the entire target population. Taking many people who propose themselves for a study results in the "self-selection bias"; they may indeed be more vigorous and healthier than the rest of the target population.

The following procedure that has sometimes been used is a good example of a bad sampling plan. In order to obtain a sample of children, one first takes a sample of households, and then *one* child from every household taken. This implies obviously that children with many sisters and brothers are underrepresented in the final sample, which results in a selection bias.

An *information bias* consists in systematic errors when measuring the exposure and outcome variables for people already in the study. This is a vast subject and we shall therefore treat it in the special Sect. 27.3.

Publication bias is something basically different from selection and information bias. It does not concern a single study but many or all studies devoted to a given problem, for instance the influence of coffee drinking on cancer of the pancreas. Thus it belongs to what is called a "meta-analysis" of results, which we shall sketch in Lesson 28. Often a publication bias arises when positive results affirming the existence of an influence of a factor are published more easily than negative ones. It is especially important in the area of clinical trials. Several thoughts may motivate a publication bias. For example the investigator may not consider negative results sufficiently interesting or useful for his career, or a clinical trial with a negative result cannot be exploited commercially.

27.3   Measurements and Quality of Data

Obtaining the data, that is measuring the values of the exposure and outcome variables for all subjects in the study population, is usually a difficult practical problem that may imply various forms of information bias. For some types of studies it is their particular structure that causes difficulties. We have for example pointed out in Sect. 20.2 that exposure variables in a case–control study concern the past and are rarely found in registers. Hence they have to be measured by asking the subjects questions like: "Did you normally drink daily more than 3 cups of vodka during the last 25 years?" They may not remember, or not want to admit that they drank much hard liquor. This gives rise to a "recall bias".

In certain sample surveys, for example in a programme like ARI (Acute Respiratory Infections) one wants to find the cause of death of a child who died without any contact with the health system; see Sects. 16.2 and 19.2. An interviewer then asks members of its family about clinical symptoms just before the moment of death in order to establish an "oral autopsy". This brings about both a recall bias and a "diagnostic bias", that is, a systematic error in the diagnosis.

Whatever the type of the study may be, leaving apart information from registers, most data are obtained by *questionnaires*. They are presented to the members of the study population by *interviewers*, either in person or via the telephone, or sent to them by mail or online. Classical questionnaires were and are on paper but electronic ones now prevail. They allow an automatic transfer of the entries into the central computer used for the statistical analysis.

A questionnaire needs to be very clearly structured, following a well-defined system and displaying easily readable captions. This is straightforward for the type of studies to which we have restricted ourselves in order to highlight the essential ideas, namely only one binary exposure variable and only one binary outcome variable. There a question about the exposure will have a "yes or no" form, to be coded by 1 and 0, respectively, and to be represented in the questionnaire by two adjacent boxes; analogously for the outcome. Such a question is a particular case of a so-called "closed" question to which only a finite number of answers, each of them corresponding to a box in the questionnaire, is possible. In an "open" or "open ended" question the person who is being interviewed formulates the answer herself or himself.

For a sample survey about many indicators, the questionnaire becomes complicated. One of the most frequent mistakes made is to put too many questions into the survey instead of restricting oneself to the really interesting and useful indicators. Too many questions are time-consuming and therefore expensive, give rise to more mistakes when filling in the questionnaires and transferring the data into the central computer and make it harder to evaluate and to present the results in lectures and publications. They also cause purely statistical problems by raising the overall error probability; see Sect. 12.4.

This problem is even more important when we conduct an epidemiologic study with many exposure or many outcome variables instead of a sample survey. The design of the questionnaire always takes much thought but it also depends a lot on the specific study at hand. Hence we shall not enter into technical details here.

The next step in order to obtain the data is to train the interviewers about how to approach the subjects in the study, how to put the questions to them, and how to fill in the questionnaires. Again, all of this depends on many specific aspects such as the socio-economic, cultural and ethnic composition of the target population and the kind of study. It would be futile to give here general rules to be learned by heart. One important aspect, however, is to make sure that all interviewers agree more or less on their way of gathering the data. This can be part of a pilot survey.

Even with a well-designed questionnaire and well-trained interviewers there usually remain mistakes in the data, that is, "measurement errors". They arise while filling in the questionnaires and while transferring the data from one medium to another one. If there is a systematic cause, this will result in a "measurement bias", which is again a particular information bias. "Misclassification" where a subject is put into the wrong category among several possible categories, for example a woman being recorded as a man, is a particular measurement bias. It can lead to a "classification bias".

Therefore the final set of data is often submitted to a check for discovering and eliminating obvious mistakes that manifest themselves in inconsistencies. Examples are a man having died of cervix cancer, a child being 77 years old, age and date of birth in contradiction. There may also be too many "outliers" (Sect. 13.2), which, although not being impossible, are highly improbable.

Finally some data may be missing. There are methods to correct for this in the final analysis by using the information contained in the existing data and perhaps other types of *a priori* information (Sect. 12.4). This is a rather difficult mathematical subject, though.

27.4 Evaluation and Interpretation

We have already observed several times that the analysis of the data from a sample survey or an epidemiologic study depends crucially on the type of investigation and in particular on the way the data have been obtained. Hence we have described their evaluation separately for each kind of study in the Lessons 12, 16–20 and 24, with examples in other lessons. It is especially important to keep this in mind when using statistical software for the analysis. The following fundamental rule is often neglected:

Never use statistical software when you don't thoroughly understand the essential aspects of your survey or study and the principles underlying the software in question.

The *interpretation* of results is relatively easy as long as we restrict ourselves to the simple studies presented in this book. It becomes less straightforward as soon as more than two exposure or outcome variables are involved. In particular, the role of confounders usually requires careful scrutiny. This is beyond the scope of the present book; some remarks can be found in Lesson 28.

27.5 Ethics

In the early times of epidemiologic studies, ethical issues used to play a minor role. It also happened that investigators circumvented them. For example they organized a study, which they could not do in their own country because of strict ethical regulations, in another country that did not impose such restrictions. Now the great importance of abiding to ethical rules is more and more being recognized.

There are two kinds of ethical issues, those concerning individuals who take part in the study, and those that bear on society. The most serious ethical issue that concerns individuals has been that of withholding a possibly beneficial preventive or curative treatment from participants in a clinical trial or community study. We have discussed it in Sects. 18.4 and 24.2. It may also happen that the treatment to be investigated is harmful to participants in a clinical trial.

We have mentioned as well the necessity of "informed consent". Any subject of the study population has to know the purpose and the main procedures of the study, thus enabling him or her in principle to judge both the value of the trial and the risks incurred.

Another ethical issue is "confidentiality". People taking part in a study must be sure that their general personal data as well as data about exposure and outcome are used only for the statistical evaluation, cannot be exploited for any other purpose and cannot be passed on to anybody outside the study. This issue becomes particularly important when studies give rise to databases in computers, which are easily accessible.

The preceding remarks concerned experimental studies. In observational studies there are no direct risks to the study population because nothing is being done to its members. However, recently another ethical problem has appeared, namely whether the information on the exposure and outcome variables obtained during the study should always be communicated to the subjects. We should normally say: "yes, why not", but in genetic epidemiology (Sect. 26.3) one has argued that knowledge by the subject of facts about her or his genome may be harmful to her or him. For example if a person in the study learns that it carries a susceptibility gene for a certain form of cancer, it may worry unnecessarily and seek superfluous or harmful treatments. The problem is related to that of "over-diagnosis" in screening; see Sect. 19.3.

In a study which concerns society as a whole the main ethical problem is that of its "quality". An ill planned or badly conducted investigation, perhaps even poorly motivated, is not only a waste of money and time but may also lead to wrong decisions of health authorities.

"Conflict of interest" is another common ethical issue. If a study is conducted or financed by an institution, for example by a commercial enterprise, that has an interest in a particular result as it is common practice in clinical trials of curative and preventive drug treatments and vaccines, a very critical appraisal by neutral scientists is indispensable. These scientists ought to obtain the complete reports on the study including the study plan and the data. However, they are not always neutral; they suffer from a conflict of interest as soon as they are not completely independent of the enterprise that did the study. For example they may receive financial or material help for their own work.

A conflict of interest can also arise if a scientist has to decide whether to launch a study that will be helpful to her or his career but is of doubtful utility. A publication bias is often the consequence of a conflict of interest. An investigator may publish only those results that are useful to him instead of publishing all results in the interest of truth.

27.6 Reading and Publishing

Searching the literature for previous results about the questions to be answered by a study is an essential part of writing the study plan. However, reading the published accounts of epidemiologic investigations also plays an important role in teaching epidemiology. Both students and people already in the health system should read and analyze a large selection of them. They should state again in their own words what the objectives and the utility were, the target population, the type of study, the indicators, the sampling procedure and the samples, the measuring methods for exposure and outcome variables, the statistical evaluation and the resulting estimated indicators, the final interpretation of the results, and perhaps recommendations for Public Health based on them.

They ought to be very critical. Were the objectives worthwhile investigating? Were all the elements above described sufficiently clearly in the article? Is there in the beginning a purely descriptive analysis where the frequency of values of the variables is given separately before the analysis of the influence of the exposures on the health variables? Is this analysis correct? Are there methodological mistakes? Is there a good distinction between essential and unessential results? Are there a good summary at the start and a concise conclusion at the end?

The reader of a study should take a particularly critical look at the bibliography. It has become fashionable to blow it up by giving references to facts that are more or less obvious and generally known. Also, very recent papers are often being quoted for results that had been published a long time ago. The authors of the present book stumbled over an article which quoted a paper that had appeared only a few years back for a result that had been known since antiquity. Generally speaking, referring to *primary* sources is preferable to using *secondary* ones.

Language and style of the publication at hand are also important elements.

Having critically read many articles about previous studies will prepare a study team to write itself a good paper about its work, taking into account the criteria above.

27.7 Practical Work

Read many accounts of epidemiologic studies of all types, both technical reports and articles in the literature.

Lesson 28
What Is Missing?

Practically all topics in epidemiology are extensions or generalizations of those treated in this book. In the present lesson we give first a short overview of extensions and generalizations of epidemiologic techniques. We then sketch the epidemiology of some more particular subject areas.

28.1 Technical Issues

In the "methodological Lessons 15–21" we have restricted ourselves to the case of only one exposure variable, which, in addition, was supposed to be binary, with the exception of Lesson 21 where we wanted the reader to understand the idea of *confounding*. However, almost all health outcomes are influenced by several factors acting together; they are "multi-factorial" and "multi-causal". For example whether a person contracts tuberculosis depends on many of the factors listed in Sects. 1.5 and 7.2 in addition to the intensity and duration of his or her exposition to the pathogen. Genetic factors play a role and so do the environment of the subject, previous infections, her or his life style and her or his social and economic standing. Often some factors "interact" with each other, which means, vaguely speaking, that their joint influence is different from the sum of their influences taken separately. In this case, each factor is called an "effect modifier" of the other ones.

In order to analyze the action of several exposure factors together we need more advanced mathematical–statistical methods. They usually rely on a "statistical model", which represents in mathematical terms certain assumptions that we make about the form of this action. Most models are "regression models". They generalize the simple regression model described in Sect. 13.3 and rely on the same basic idea. These general models also allow us to analyze exposure and outcome variables that are no longer binary but either continuous or categorical with more than two categories; see Sect. 13.1.

The investigation of complex situations often requires "study designs" beyond the simple designs treated in Lessons 15–20.

An important omission in this book has been the time dimension of events. "Time" has appeared only in a few places. In its simplest form, it enters the concept

© Springer Nature Switzerland AG 2019
K. Krickeberg et al., *Epidemiology*, Statistics for Biology and Health,
https://doi.org/10.1007/978-3-030-16368-6_28

of a "rate". Generally speaking a rate is a number of events per unit of time. For example an incidence rate is sometimes defined as the number of new cases of a given disease in the target population per unit of time. Care needs to be taken not to confuse this with the definition given in Sect. 15.1 where incidence rate was identified with incidence density, that is, the number of new cases divided by the size of the target population.

"Longitudinal studies", mentioned briefly at the end of Sect. 16.2, would also deserve a more detailed treatment.

Time is the essential dimension in the so-called "survival analysis". There we are dealing with outcome variables that represent "waiting times", for example the survival time of cancer patients after chemotherapy. Their study is nowadays an important part of clinical trials.

"Meta-analysis" was mentioned in Sect. 27.2. It means evaluating many or all studies devoted to a given problem in order to reach an overall conclusion. Such an evaluation will involve comparing the studies at hand and trying to synthesize their results. Different studies of the same problem do not always use the same concepts and methods, though. Their design, sample sizes, definition of variables and many other elements may be very different. Each study is subject to many mistakes such as random errors due to small samples or wrong sampling methods, various forms of bias, faulty handling of confounders etc. Hence it is indeed tempting to "pool" studies in order to reach more reliable results. However, synthesizing their conclusions rigorously requires fairly sophisticated mathematical–statistical tools due to the different nature of the studies. Many so-called "survey articles"which only list and discuss various published studies are wrongly called meta-analyses.

Elements of the *history* of epidemiology appear in several places of this book including the Lesson 29 below. A systematic and comprehensive history of our field from its beginnings still needs to be written.

28.2 Epidemiology of Some More Particular Subject Areas

The "missing" topics listed in the preceding section all belong to what is called "general" epidemiology, whose concepts and methods apply to all kinds of exposure and health outcomes. The reader has no doubt noticed, and we have said it before, that some of the "special" topics treated in the present text are defined by a particular *outcome*. This is true for those of Lessons 3, 6–10, 22 and 23. In contrast to that the subject of Lessons 25 and 26 is determined by a particular kind of *exposure*.

There exist of course many more special topics. They may be determined by other diseases as outcomes. For example the epidemiology of arthrosis and other degenerative ailments would be particularly important for Vietnam. Regarding issues defined by input variables we have for instance the risk factors aging, work stress, more life style factors such as physical exercise, and malpractice of a doctor. The books of the series "Basic Texts in Public Health" listed at the end of the Preface also provide many more details of epidemiologic topics.

28.3   Practical Work

Leaf through the whole book again, reflect on the various topics, and decide what are, in your opinion, the most useful elements for the health of the population.

Lesson 29
The Role of Epidemiology in Building Coherent Systems of Public Health

Public Health is not a collection of various dispersed services of the health system of a country. It is a clearly defined large subject area like pharmacy or medicine. It needs to be built by developing its components in a coherent way. This process rests on research, teaching and practical experiences like those sketched in the preceding lessons.

29.1 Understanding Public Health

In most if not all countries of the world Public Health is being built and operated in a piecemeal way. Its various parts are rarely linked to each other by an all-embracing concept and often not by their practice either. The reasons are largely historical. A particular Public Health Service was created when there seemed to be a more or less urgent need. Screening in schools for tooth decay, bad eyesight and other ailments is a typical example. This practice started about one and a half centuries ago. Preventive measures such as hygiene, clean drinking water, sewage systems, and recommendations about nutrition and physical activities are documented from ancient Egypt, China, Greece and Rome but not as parts of a general systematic effort. Immunizations followed in the nineteenth Century after some forerunners; see Sect. 5.1.

Public Health as an entire system of measures emerged in the nineteenth Century. It was mostly called Social Hygiene but the term Public Health, too, appeared soon, in particular in 1848 in the "Public Health Act" of the United Kingdom (see Sect. 26.1). At present it seems that all or almost all languages of the world use a literal or slightly elaborated translation of this term. The authors of the present book have verified it for the following languages or groups of languages: Vietnamese; Chinese; Arabian; Hebrew; Turkish; Hungarian; Greek; Slavonic; Romance; Germanic.

However, to employ a largely accepted term does not mean to understand it. The main obstacle to an understanding was the profusion of definitions given, starting with one proposed at the end of the 1980s. All of them consisted of an enumeration of particular health services, but they varied between definitions by different persons or organizations and occasionally even between several definitions stated by the same organization at different times.

© Springer Nature Switzerland AG 2019

K. Krickeberg et al., *Epidemiology*, Statistics for Biology and Health,

https://doi.org/10.1007/978-3-030-16368-6_29

A second obstacle was due to the lack of understanding of Public Health by the majority of physicians. Their organizations usually tried and are trying to dominate the entire Health System and to regard and treat Public Health as a small and not very important sub-area of medicine. This state of affairs varies a lot between countries. In Vietnam it is still visible but relatively minor.

We have given an unambiguous definition of Public Health in the very first Section of this book. It is short and easy to understand, and does not need to be changed in the course of time. Our 2nd lesson shows that it covers indeed the topics that have normally been considered to belong to Public Health. The example of Genetic Epidemiology (Lesson 26) proves that it is also the right frame for certain new issues that may be regarded as part of Public Health.

All of these topics and areas rely heavily on epidemiologic methods. From the point of view of the practice of Public Health we might even employ the following alternative definition:

Public Health is Applied Epidemiology.

29.2   First Structural and Administrative Steps

From prehistoric times until a few centuries ago there were only few structures or administrations for Public Health. They dealt with water supply, bathing facilities and sewage but also with some forms of hygiene. For example during the Vietnamese Later Lê Dynasty, which began in 1427, slaughterhouses and the sale of meat were controlled by health officials. In some countries administrations and institutions such as religious groups built public hospitals.

In the late 18th and early nineteenth Century many ideas and proposals for providing Public Health activities within an administrative frame appeared, mainly in Europe and the USA. However, one should rather say "providing Public Health activities with *many* administrative frames" because there was no unifying concept. Administrations of cities, regions and countries set up departments that were usually meant for special tasks.

The most systematic and extended measures for structuring Public Health came mainly from universities, starting in the second half of the nineteenth Century. They took two forms. Firstly, Universities established Chairs, Departments or Schools of Hygiene, mostly within a Faculty of Medicine. Secondly, university professors and lecturers together with their physician colleagues in various medical institutions wrote extensively about their new ideas on Social Hygiene, also called Social Health, and translated them into practical work.

The University Departments or Schools of Hygiene had a clearly defined objective from their beginning, namely prevention of infectious diseases. Many of them are still doing only that. In addition, more specialized ones appeared, for example Schools of Dental Hygiene. The groups of people promoting Social Hygiene were working in a different setting, taking social and economic factors into account. The range of their activities was also wider, including for instance, in addition to personal hygiene, screening programmes and systematic treatment of some health defects.

The next steps were taken from the early twentieth Century on by founding Schools of Public Health. Several countries did so; the Hanoi School of Public Health was established in the year 2001. Their curricula usually cover the topics treated in the present book. They also intervene in various ways in the practice of the health system, for instance by research, by publishing advice on matters of health, and by counselling health institutions. However, this is hardly ever being done systematically within a well-defined wide range structure.

29.3   The Present Vietnamese System of Public Health

Some countries have built more complete and well-structured Public Health systems; Vietnam is among them. We are going to describe the Vietnamese system briefly. It comprises the Hanoi University of Public Health, which we have already mentioned, and the Vietnamese Public Health Association, which carries out specific actions in many provinces of the country.

Two further types of Public Health structures are interwoven with medical structures; this is in fact their most distinctive feature. Let us look at the details of both types and start with the first one. It is located in universities.

As in other countries, many general universities in Vietnam have a Faculty of Medicine but there are also specialized Universities of Medicine, usually combined with Pharmacy. In order to simplify our exposition we shall use the term "Faculty of Medicine" in both cases. Now:

Every Vietnamese Faculty of Medicine has a Department of Public Health. The curricula for the basic 6 years studies of Medicine include a substantial number of modules that belong partly or entirely to Public Health.

This is no doubt a great achievement.

In addition to training future physicians in Public Health many Faculties of Medicine also offer programmes to form specialists of Public Health, for example on the Bachelor and Master level.

The second kind of Public Health structure interwoven with medical ones is tied to Primary Health Structures. In Vietnam Primary Health means essentially the network of Commune Health Stations and equivalent health facilities. In addition to curative and obstetrical work they are entrusted with several Public Health activities, which we have described in many parts of the present book, in particular in the Sects. 1.2, 3.2, 4.5, 11.1, 11.2, 11.3 and 19.1. Health education of the population and implementing health programmes such as systematic immunizations are the main ones. Having created this "dual function" network for Primary Health is another great achievement.

Thus the concept of the Vietnamese Public Health System was quite good. There remained many imperfections in the details, though. Therefore, a research programme took place in the years 2006–2016 in order to analyze these flaws and to propose better structures. The main tools of this programme were yearly rotating workshops in the Medical Faculties outside of the cities of Hanoi and Ho Chi Minh-City. Thus most of their lecturers could participate at least once and many did it several times. We worked in small groups as well as in plenary sessions. Field trips to primary and district level health facilities were always included. Between the workshops we studied many problems through e-mail. The following section will present the main results.

29.4   A Coherent System of Public Health

Recall again that the following proposals are meant to serve as an example. It should not be too difficult to adapt them to other countries.

We decided at the beginning not to work with the Medical Universities of Hanoi and Ho Chi Minh-City. The man-made conditions that influence human health in the Vietnamese provinces outside of these two big cities are sufficiently different from those within them to warrant a research programme of their own. This is obviously true for environmental conditions but we are interested in conditions determined by the health system, for example the availability and quality of hospital services. Some components of the health system in these provinces are indeed not as much developed as in Hanoi and Ho Chi Minh-City; hence they need special attention.

Our point of departure was the structure of the Vietnamese Public Health System as described in the preceding section. We rapidly realized that we had to address the following issues:

1. To improve the content of teaching Public Health in the Medical Faculties.
2. To reorganize its curricula.
3. To bring the qualification and standing of the lecturers of Public Health up to level expected of lecturers of Clinical Medicine.
4. To develop clear guidelines for the functions and places of work of personnel qualified in Public Health.
5. To outline ways of providing clinical physicians with reliable and easily available information about the efficacy and side effects of their diagnostic and curative methods.
6. To plan and to monitor preventive measures.
7. To build a good health information system.
8. To create a general coherent system of health information and health competence of the population.

In the following we shall elaborate on each issue while sticking to the most essential features.

About 1 We soon discovered that the majority of textbooks used by the lecturers to inform themselves and their students were not optimal. Apart from many flaws of content and presentation they did not take the Vietnamese context into account. We therefore started the book series "Basic Texts In Public Health" sketched at the end of the Preface. Together, these texts are meant to cover the essential branches of Public Health in a coherent way, in the setting of Vietnam as an example. Important elements of the history of epidemiology appear in many places.

The publisher distributes our books to the libraries of the universities that have a Medical Faculty and to many other institutions.

About 2 This, too, concerns both the curricula of the part "Public Health" in the study course for future physicians and those for future Public Health specialists. We found that the order in which the various modules are being taught was often quite illogical. For instance modules on epidemiology appeared very late, probably because the authors of the curricula had in mind only epidemiologic study methods and not epidemiology as a whole. Some important subjects were missing, others seemed to be superfluous.

The most important missing part was a clear comparative survey of the epidemiology of infectious and of non-infectious diseases. When teaching these two areas their basic difference needs to be stressed (see Sect. 2.3). Also missing was clinical epidemiology, social epidemiology, and the history of Public Health. The problem of subject-areas that comprise both a microbiological and a population-based part, namely immunology and genetics, was ignored. These subjects might be taught to students of Medicine and students of Public Health together as a single module. Likewise a joint module on the history of both Medicine and Public Health would be highly desirable.

About 3 In all workshops all of us agreed on the following measures. Persons who apply for admission to such and such study course in Public Health (see the following paragraph no. 4) must be as qualified as future students of Medicine. In particular the common practice of redirecting to studying Public Health the applicants who failed the entrance examination to medical studies, is absurd and harmful to the health of the population. Also, lecturers of Public Health in Medical Faculties need to be as qualified as lecturers of Medicine. Their teaching load must not be higher than that of the latter and they ought to have comparable possibilities of doing research and practical work. The two categories of lecturers have to receive the same salaries.

About 4 There is still a profusion of study courses and degrees in Public Health. The following set seems to be reasonable: Bachelor of Public Health; Master of Public Health; Doctor of Public Health (the counterpart of the Doctor of General Medicine); Ph. D. in Public Health. Their functions and places of work will by and large correspond to their level. For example a nurse in a Commune Health Station or a hospital may acquire the degree of Bachelor of Public Health and a scientist who plans a large clinical trial ought to be a Ph. D. in Public Health. The Ministry of Health will make these general principles known but the actual workplace of an individual person will in general be determined by this person and by the institution which intends to employ her or him.

About 5 This will of course be a very large and never ending enterprise. It means to scrutinize the available literature in order to find out which methods are "evidence-based" (see Sect. 18.3), to initiate and implement clinical trials if necessary, to organize the dissemination and easy accessibility of the information obtained, and to make sure it is well used.

Knowledge about side effects is often as important as knowledge about efficacy. Let us quote an indirect side effect, namely the surge of bacteria that became resistant against the antibiotics that were originally used to eliminate them. The observations by Alexander Fleming in 1928 had led to the discovery of Penicillin, and antibiotics appeared on the general drug market after the Second World War. Fleming warned already in the year 1945 that misuse of Penicillin may make the microbes in question resistant but these warnings were for a long time ignored, largely to the profit of the drug industry. Now the so-called multidrug resistance is a common phenomenon, for example among *Mycobacterium tuberculosis* that causes tuberculosis and among *staphylococcus aureus* that causes some types of pneumonia. We shall not enter here the well-known details of the genesis and implications of this phenomenon; they can be found in the book on Environmental Health mentioned at the end of the Preface, Sects. 3.3 and 7.3. Ignoring it deliberately may very well be called a crime against humanity.

About 6 Preventive measures have been taken in Vietnam for a long time in many ways; they are described in many lessons of the present book. However, the basic difference between prevention of infectious and of non-infectious diseases has hardly played a role. In "About 2" above we have stressed the need to take it into account when teaching prevention, but this need exists as well when taking preventive measures in practice.

About 7 We have described the heavy faults of the various present Vietnamese Health Information Systems and the principles of a good one in Lesson 11. This analysis was refined at our workshops and published. Let us only mention two of these principles. Firstly, health information produced in a health facility, for example in a Commune Health Station, is not only meant to be reported to higher-level health offices but also to be used at the facility itself. Secondly, in a health facility there should be only one register for a given target population, in other words, never divide registers concerning the same units, for example births, into registers of different types of data, for example prenatal examinations on the one hand and diseases of the infants on the other.

About 8 This, too, will be a very large and never ending enterprise, resembling task no. 5. Some aspects were described in the books on Health Education and Nutrition mentioned in the Preface but for most of the work clear guidelines are still missing.

29.5   Practical Work for Non-Vietnamese Readers

Reread the preceding sections of the present lesson and try to imagine how you would write them if they concerned your own country.

Author Index

by Section

© Springer Nature Switzerland AG 2019
K. Krickeberg et al., *Epidemiology*, Statistics for Biology and Health,
https://doi.org/10.1007/978-3-030-16368-6

Subject Index

by Section

Printed in the United States
By Bookmasters